HERBS FOR HEALTH AND BE

MARGARET ROBERTS HERB SERIES

Herbs for Health and Beauty

Illustrated by
Sanmarie Harms

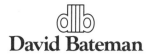

David Bateman

© Margaret Roberts 1986

Originally published by Lowry Publishers.
This edition published in 1988 by David Bateman Ltd,
'Golden Heights', 32–34 View Road, Glenfield,
Auckland 10, New Zealand

Reprinted 1989
Reprinted 1990
Reprinted 1992

ISBN 1 86953 006 3

A David Bateman book
Printed in Hong Kong by Colorcraft

Contents

Introduction

The hectic pace at which most of us live our lives takes its toll on our faces and our bodies. Stress, anxiety, tension – these are words and conditions with which we have become all too familiar. Most of us are ageing far faster than we ought to be.

There is no doubt that beauty shines from within and no body or facial preparation can replace the true contentment of a serene and peaceful mind. The aim of this little book is to put serenity and calmness back into strained faces, a shine back into limp, dull hair, relaxation into tension-filled shoulders, and peace into taut minds.

It is said that what we put into life is what we'll get out of it. And so it is with our bodies: we can do much to improve our mental and physical health by using only pure, natural ingredients, both internally and externally. Herbs are natural beautifiers and in turning these pages you will be able to share with me my own health and beauty secrets.All these preparations have been tried and tested, used and enjoyed over many years. I hope that they will give you the pleasure and wonderful results they have given me.

My thanks go to those who have supported and criticised, sampled and experimented, encouraged and delighted in this fascinating subject. May you always remain beautiful! Thank you, too, to June Jackson and Kathrine Marais for their expert deciphering and typing, to Sanmarie Harms for her exquisite illustrations, and to my editor, Alison Lowry, who manages to get everything in order.

Herbs for Health and Beauty is my gift to all who want to use their green heritage to its best advantage.

1

How to Prepare Herbs

In making up the simple recipes used in this book there are various methods of preparing herbs for use in lotions and creams. The methods listed below will help you to get started.

Decoction

A decoction of herb usually means the boiling up of the herb, and it is usually prepared by using roots, stems, bark and berries, ie the hard parts of plants. The herb or part of the herb is boiled for about 15 minutes and then allowed to cool. The resulting liquid is drawn off and used and the herb is discarded.

Infusion

When you pour boiling water over a herb (fresh or dried) and leave it to stand for about 15 minutes, this is known as an infusion. The same method is used to make *herbal tea*, and the strained 'tea' is the part used. The herb is discarded.

Cold Infusion

In a cold infusion the herb is allowed to steep in a cold liquid such as vinegar or oil, wine or alcohol. It should be allowed a longer period to stand, and should be placed in a sealed, airtight container.

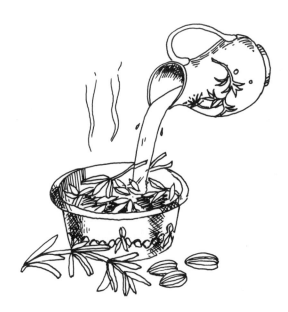

Essential Oil

Besides their healing properties, essential oils add fragrance to a cream or lotion. With a little extra trouble you can prepare your own oils. Particularly in making cosmetics, natural ingredients will enhance your beauty preparations and are infinitely preferable. The essential oils available commercially are of necessity synthetic. We would never be able to afford the real oil of a flower as several tons of petals go into the making of one cup of true flower oil. This recipe is the next best thing, and it is quick and easy to make.

I always use fresh herbs as their fragrance and active principles are then at their best. If you are unable to obtain fresh herbs, however, dried herbs will do as well. Merely halve the quantities, ie 250 ml (1 cup) fresh to 125 ml (½ cup) dried herb.

250 ml (1 cup) fresh chopped herbs
500 ml (2 cups) vegetable oil, eg maize, sunflower or almond oil
12,5 ml (1 tbsp) apple cider vinegar

3

Pour into a screw-top jar, shake vigorously and place in the sun. Let the oil mature for a week to 10 days. Shake each day. Then strain through cheesecloth or a nylon sieve, using a wooden spoon. Repeat the process, using fresh herbs, until the aroma is strong enough for your liking. Finally strain and pour into dark glass bottles. Date and label the bottles.

Tincture

A tincture is made with medicinal alcohol or, if you cannot get it, vodka is available from all bottle-stores. Steep 100 g dried herb (or 200 g fresh herb) in 1 litre (4 cups) alcohol for 2 weeks, in a screw-top jar. Shake daily. Filter before using it, and always keep the bottle tightly sealed.

Water

When water is called for in a recipe, try to use distilled water as hard water can have a harsh effect on your skin. Fresh rain-water is also preferable.

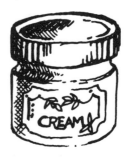

Herb Creams

These can be simply made by pounding a quantity of fresh herbs directly into the creams. Lots of pounding and energy is required. Use a pestle and mortar or a liquidiser. Petroleum jelly is a good base or an aqueous cream, available from most pharmacies.

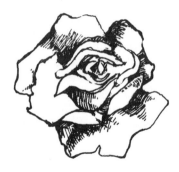

Herb Milk

Milk readily absorbs the oils from herbs and the preparation is easy. Use 250 ml (1 cup) chopped fresh herb to 500 ml (2 cups) milk. Mix well, cover and stand for about 4 hours. (In mid-summer's heat I keep the mixture in the fridge.) Then strain through a fine sieve, mashing out the juices with a wooden spoon. Rose petals and calendula petals can be used this way and lemon balm, rosemary and lavender leaves are particularly pleasant. The milk can be used for cleansing, tightening the pores and as a soothing sunburn treatment.

Maceration (Wine)

Both red and white wine can be used, but I find white wine kinder to tender skin. Here you will need 250–500 ml (1–2 cups) fresh herb leaves to 1 litre (4 cups) wine. Dried bark, seeds or berries can also be used, but bruise them first in a pestle and mortar. Leave for 3 days, then strain. A little of this mixture taken internally every now and then can only be good for you, particularly if you have used rosemary, elder berries, or lavender. Used as a cosmetic, it is astringent and toning.

Maceration (Vinegar)

The ideal vinegar for cosmetic purposes is apple cider vinegar as it helps restore the acid mantle your skin so badly needs. It is good for softening rough, flaky skin and soothing itchiness.

Herb vinegar is easy to make. Take a bottle of apple cider vinegar and empty out a little (save it for your bath). Press in as much herb as you can get into the bottle. Place the bottle in the sun. After 3 or 4 days replace the herb with fresh herb. Do this 2 or 4 times, following the same procedure. Finally strain and bottle in a dark glass bottle. Label and date carefully.

Herbs that particularly lend themselves to vinegars are lavender, rosemary, scented geranium, yarrow, lemon verbena, rose (petals), calendula, mint, sage, eucalyptus, bergamot, catmint, lemon thyme, and lemon balm.

Compresses

For some skin cleansing and healing processes, a compress is an ideal way of stimulating circulation to relieve muscular aches and pains. Essentially a compress is merely a face-cloth or towel wrung out in a strong, hot decoction or infusion, and applied to the area, held in place for a time and then repeated as desired. Hot and cold compresses can be alternated. Do not use compresses if you have thread veins on your face, however, and if you have a dry skin massage a little almond oil into it first. Cold compresses soothe puffiness, and reduce large pores, swelling and bruises.

Poultices

Poultices are an effective treatment, directly applied, for stubborn blackheads, boils or spots. Use the actual herb, warmed and softened in boiling water, holding it in place for a few minutes. This can be repeated 2 or 3 times, using fresh herb each time. Geranium leaves, comfrey leaves, yarrow and pawpaw leaves are all excellent.

Facial Skin Care

PATCH TEST

Before starting your herbal treatments always do a patch test. Dab a little of your preparation on the pulse point of your wrist or in the crook of your elbow. Leave it unwashed for 12 hours to see whether you have an allergic reaction to it. Always be sure of the identification of the herbs you are using and if ever you are in doubt, consult your doctor or skin specialist. Many people are allergic to a wide range of ingredients and I urge you to tread with care and always test your blends and mixtures, lotions and salves before using them.

CLEANSING

There are literally hundreds of creams, lotions, tonics and soaps available on the market, enough to confuse anyone. I like to keep my cosmetics simple and effective and the following is a list of natural facial cleansers, fresh and delightful to use, and available to all at very little cost.

Rainwater

The softest and most beautiful water of all – perfect for washing the face and hair. Make a plan to catch some, in a big clean basin, next time it rains.

Buttermilk

Fresh buttermilk can be patted and massaged into the skin. It will tighten pores and tone the skin, as well as cleanse thoroughly. Rinse with clean, clear water.

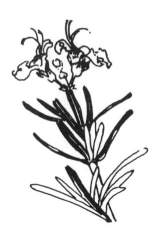

Herb Milk

Take a cup of chopped rosemary, comfrey, violets, sage, lavender, or scented geranium. Mix into 500 ml (2 cups) fresh milk. Stand for about 4 hours (in the refrigerator in summer), then strain and store in the refrigerator. Use the milk to cleanse the skin, using pads of cottonwool. Even when it thickens it can still be used. I make small quantities frequently.

Cucumber

Next time you make a salad, save the skins of the cucumbers. Use them to clean the face, discarding after use. Alternatively, mash up cucumber pulp, 125 ml (½ cup) pulp, with 25 ml (2 tbsp) milk. Store what you don't use in the refrigerator.

Oatmeal

Make a paste out of oatmeal which has been soaked overnight in water. I find the large flake (non-instant) oatmeal best for this. Use a handful of the mixture as a scrub. Mixed with a strong comfrey leaf infusion instead of water, and left to soften overnight, it is healing for acne, excellent for getting rid of

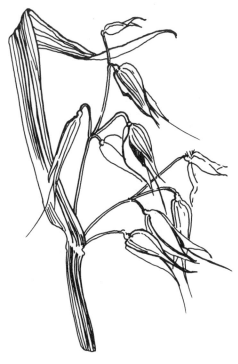

spots and pimples on the back and neck, and soothing for sunburn. Use 250 ml (1 cup) chopped comfrey to 500 ml (2 cups) boiling water. Stand for 20 minutes, then pour off the tea. Add to this 1 cup of oats. Cover and leave to stand overnight. Use to wash and scrub the face, neck and back each evening.

Rosewater

Distilled and bottled rosewater can be bought from chemists. Alternatively, you can make your own: use 6 cups red rose petals to 1 litre (4 cups) water (preferably rainwater). Boil up for 15 minutes. Cool, strain, bottle and keep in the refrigerator.

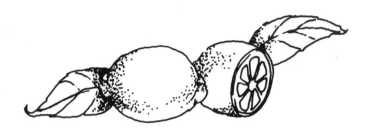

Lemon

Lemon juice is antiseptic and cleansing and restores the acidity of the skin. Excellent for the prevention of blackheads, lemon juice can also be used combined with a variety of herbs. Use the skins of squeezed lemons to clean nails and dingy skin on elbows and knees.

Soapwort

Soothing and healing, a strong brew can be made from soapwort (*Saponaria officinalis*) by boiling up a potful of roots, stems, flowers and leaves with enough water to cover. Boil for 10 minutes, stand, cool and strain. It can be used as a face wash, a hair wash and hair conditioner, and can also be dabbed onto eczema.

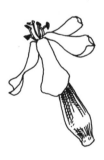

Tomato and Lemon Oily Skin Cleanser

Both tomato and lemon are astringent and nourishing for the skin. Chop up, roughly, 1 medium-sized ripe tomato and squeeze out the juice. Add the pulp of 1 lemon. Liquidise for 2–3 minutes. Spread this thin paste on the face, working it in gently with the fingers. Wash off with tepid water. This is an excellent cleanser for oily skin and should be applied two or three times a week. Save any excess and store in the refrigerator.

Herbal Steam Cleansers

Particularly good in a Mediterranean-type climate, herbal steam cuts down external grease and deep cleanses the pores.
If you have thread veins in your face, however, you should avoid steaming. In a large bowl place ½ cup of one or two of the following herbs: elder flowers, chamomile leaves and flowers, scented geranium leaves, lavender leaves and flowers, rosemary leaves and flowers, yarrow leaves and flowers, peppermint sprigs, eucalyptus leaves. Pour 500–750 ml (2–3 cups) boiling water over the herb. Improvise a towel tent and hold your face over the bowl for about 7–10 minutes. Pat dry, then splash or dab on an astringent to close the pores.

Soap

Always choose a pure soap for your face. Chemists offer a range of excellent beauty soaps – aloe vera and herbs, honey and goatsmilk, buttermilk and cucumber. It is largely a matter of personal choice. Select with care the best for your skin and ask the pharmacist for advice if you are hesitant.

Cleansing Cream

If you use heavy make-up you will need a heavy cream to remove it, particularly in the case of eye make-up. The following is a simple recipe that is pure and natural. It costs very little to make and is just as good as the more expensive creams on the market. It also makes an excellent night cream.

1 measure anhydrous lanolin
3 measures almond oil
1 measure rosewater (available from chemists)
½ measure water soluble cream, eg aqueous cream

In a double boiler slowly melt together the lanolin and the soluble cream, stirring all the time. Add the almond oil and the rosewater. Remove from heat. Pour the mixture into an opaque jar. A few drops of flower oil can be added as it cools to give it an aroma, but this is optional.

Vaseline Cleansing Cream

15 g white vaseline
15 g beeswax
50 g almond oil
20 g rosewater

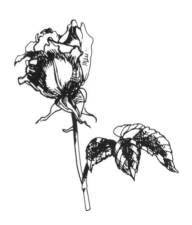

Heat the vaseline and beeswax in a double boiler. Heat the rosewater and almond oil over a low heat. Remove from the heat and combine by adding a little of the rosewater and almond oil mixture to the melted vaseline and beeswax, whisking all the time. Continue whisking until it cools. Half a cup calendula petals infused in 125 ml (½ cup) boiling water can be added to the almond oil and rosewater to make a pouring cream (strain before adding to the lanolin and beeswax). Pour into screw-top jars. Label and date.

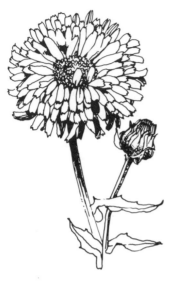

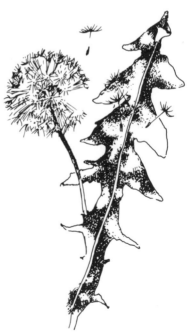

PROBLEM SKIN: PIMPLES, SPOTS, ACNE

The most important aspect of skin care is diet. Drink lots of water, eat plenty of fresh fruit and vegetables, and avoid fatty, fried foods, chocolate and refined sugars, flours, carbonated drinks, coffee, peanuts and iodised salt. Fresh salads daily, with lots of green, chlorophyll-rich ingredients in it, are essential.

There are certain herbs known as depuratives, which cleanse the system by purifying the blood, and this in turn helps ensure a clear skin. Borage and watercress are two depuratives, lemons and oranges are another two. Four common weeds which make excellent blood cleansers are plantain, chickweed, sow's thistle and dandelion. The young leaves of these weeds can be finely chopped and added to salads. Also effective are infusions, which can be drunk or used as a wash. Lavender, calendula petals, sage, borage leaves and flowers, and dandelion leaves can all be used – 60 ml (¼ cup) herb to 250 ml (1 cup) boiling water.

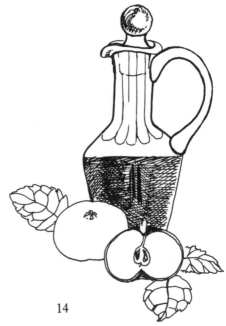

Apple Cider Vinegar

Apple cider vinegar is a wonderful wash for problem skins as it helps to combat oiliness. Dilute 60 ml (¼ cup) vinegar to 750 ml (3 cups) tepid water and use as a wash, or drink a little every day: 1–2 teaspoons in a glass of tepid water. This is, incidentally, a wonderful cooling revitalizer in the heat of summer, particularly after vigorous exercise. It can also be used as a compress, held over bad spots or dabbed onto the affected area. Dilute to the strength most acceptable to your needs. Many people find it too strong to apply neat.

Blackhead Remover

Herbal steam cleansers soften and penetrate, facilitating the removal of blackheads. Make a hot herbal infusion, using yarrow, comfrey, or nettle, with a little apple cider vinegar. Pat almond oil onto the blackheads. Soak a towel in the hot infusion, wring out and apply several times as the towel cools. Then gently push out the blackheads. *NB. Always be sure your hands and nails are scrupulously clean when touching spots on your face.*

Blemish Controllers

Fresh cucumber juice or slices, crushed watercress leaves or juice, and crushed sow's thistle leaves or juice are all excellent blemish controllers. Pat onto the affected area and leave overnight. Wash off next morning with clean, clear water. Another effective method is to make a decoction of myrtle leaves and rue flowers. Pat on, and leave overnight. Alternatively, make a paste using grated fresh horse-radish root mixed with a little apple cider vinegar, or elder flowers crushed with a little lemon juice. Smear onto the area and leave for 15–20 minutes. Wash off with a gentle astringent.

Brown Spots

Liver spots or age spots are often attributed to lack of vitamins B, E and C. It is unwise to treat yourself in this case as too much of a vitamin is as bad as too little, and you should rather consult your doctor. Include the following vitamin-rich foods in your diet:

Vitamin B: debittered Torula yeast (use in gravies, soups and stews), liver, wheatgerm, green peas, sunflower seeds, brown rice, eggs, lentils, soyabeans, bananas, raisins, yoghurt, cream cheese.

Vitamin C: oranges, lemons, mandarins, grapefruit, guavas, pineapple, green peppers, tomato, cabbage.

Vitamin E: Wheatgerm oil, nuts, dairy products, leafy greens.

An old folk remedy is gently to massage castor oil into brown spots, and some people claim that this is indeed effective.

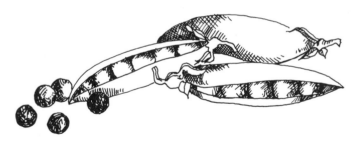

ASTRINGENTS

Astringents are pore closers and have a bracing and toning effect on the skin. They contract the skin, tightening and drying it. Astringents should be used after deep cleansing and steaming.

Cucumber

This everyday vegetable is a natural astringent – and incidentally contains an 'anti-wrinkle' hormone.

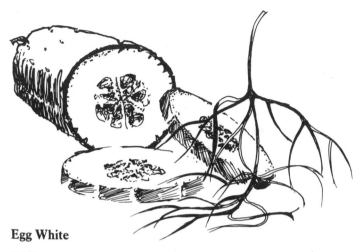

Egg White

Stiffly whisked egg white is a wonderful astringent. Pat on after deep cleansing the skin, and leave for 15 minutes. Wash off with clear, tepid water.

Strawberry

Excellent for reducing oiliness and bracing and toning the skin. Mash and apply to the face for a marvellous home facial.

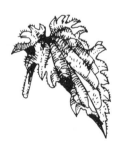

Herb Decoctions

For *oily skin:* yarrow, chamomile
For *combination skin:* sage, nettle

Boil up 1 cup leaves and flowers of herb in 1 litre (4 cups) water. Simmer for 5 minutes. Remove from the stove, cover and allow to cool. Strain off and bottle the liquid. Keep refrigerated.

Body Beautiful

HANDS AND FEET

We may admire the man with strong, work-hardened, calloused hands, but no matter how hard a woman works, no matter her age, she is expected to have soft, smooth, well cared for hands at all times. Cook, gardener, housewife, mother, repairman, painter, and bottle-washer – the woman of today does it all and to keep her hands and her feet beautiful is pretty hard to achieve.

Through the years I have worked out a few beauty aids that have stood the test of time, and these I share with you in the hope that they will prove as rewarding to you as they have to me.

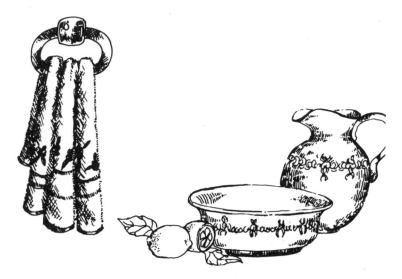

Protection for Hands

Consider first the lowly lemon, one of my favourite fruits. Its place in natural cosmetics is paramount. The lemon serves as a whitener, skin softener, cuticle softener and remover, nail cleaner, smell and stain remover, and skin toner, restoring the acid coating the skin needs.

Once you have used lemon juice in cooking, save the squeezed halves. Dig your nails into it and rub the pulp and skin all over your hands, or feet, paying particular attention to rough heels. You can use up every bit of its goodness. Massage your feet with the skin, and rub the inner white pith over your nails, softening the cuticles.

Lemon Brandy Hand Lotion

This is a very old softening and soothing lotion for rough, chapped hands. It keeps well, too, as the brandy preserves it.

125 ml (½ cup) freshly squeezed lemon juice
125 ml (½ cup) white wine vinegar in which a few sprigs of basil have been steeped
250 ml (1 cup) brandy

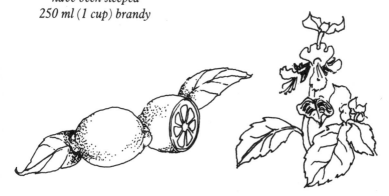

Shake all the ingredients together in a screw-top jar. Keep beside the basin in the bathroom and apply frequently to hands after washing.

Protective Barrier Cream

This is an excellent cream to use before gardening or any manual work. Make a fresh batch each time and you will find it very effective.

1 dessertspoon kaolin (white powdered clay, or Fuller's earth,
available from chemists)
10 ml (2 tsp) almond oil
1 egg yolk

Whisk up all ingredients and rub into the hands, working under the nails and massaging deep into the skin. Allow to dry. When you come in from the garden, wash it off, and you'll be amazed at how soft your skin is. It is also excellent for feet, particularly if you are gardening barefoot or in sandals.

Glove Treatment

This is the most softening and conditioning of all treatments, but, as you are supposed to wear them overnight, the sight of gloves oozing herbs and oatmeal could be grounds for divorce! Buy a pair of cotton gloves, a size or two too big for you. You will also need a large pair of plastic disposable gloves to fit over your paste-filled cotton gloves to protect the sheets. Make up the 'pomade' as follows:

125 ml (1/2 cup) almonds
250 ml (1 cup) boiling water
1 egg, beaten
12,5 ml (1 tbsp) honey
few drops almond oil

Pour the water over the almonds to loosen the skin. Stand for a few minutes, then drain off the water, skin the almonds and pulverise. Add egg, honey and a few drops of almond oil.

Spread the mixture all over your hands and ask someone to help you put on your gloves. Tie at the wrists, not too tightly but enough to prevent the plastic gloves from sliding off. Sleep with the gloves on and you will be astounded at how beautiful your skin feels in the morning once you've washed off the paste.

Chapped Hand Glove

125 ml (½ cup) finely chopped or minced borage leaves
1 dessertspoon castor oil
125 ml (½ cup) oats
1 dessertspoon honey

Mix into a paste, adding a little hot water to the borage leaves. Spread over the hands, put on the gloves and keep them on for an hour or two, or overnight.

Hard Skin Softener

Mix a tablespoon of coarse sea salt with a tablespoon of almond oil, and rub vigorously into the hard, horny areas. Then hop into a bath, adding a little more oil to the bathwater, and soak the well-rubbed areas for at least 10 minutes. Then rub the hard skin away with a pumice stone. After your bath soothe the worked area with a good cream or lotion.

Mask for Horny Skin

This is particularly good for roughened hands and heels.

2–4 cups soapwort, flowers, roots and leaves, steeped in 2
*   litres (8 cups) boiling water*
250 ml (1 cup) pawpaw, mashed OR
2–3 slices pineapple, mashed
half an avocado
250–500 ml (1–2 cups) bran
4 scented geranium leaves, minced

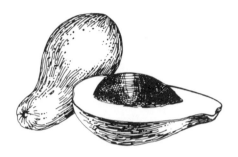

Mash all the ingredients together, except soapwort, adding enough bran to make the mixture adhere. Soak hands or feet in the soapwort brew for 10 minutes. Dry the skin. Spread the mask on hands or feet in a thick layer. Leave on for 20 minutes, then wash off in the soapwort brew, using a pumice stone. Rub a good cream into the area.

NB Never pare off horny skin with a razor blade. Rather use a pumice stone.

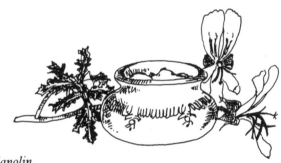

Hand Cream

25 ml (2 tbsp) lanolin
12,5 ml (1 tbsp) liquid paraffin
25 ml (2 tbsp) herbal infusion, eg scented geranium, lavender, camphor leaves, eucalyptus leaves, basil, elder (250 ml (1 cup) herb to 500 ml (2 cups) boiling water; stand, steep, cool, strain)
37,5 ml (3 tbsp) aqueous cream

Whisk all ingredients together. Store in a screw-top jar. Use lavishly on dry hands. It is also good for dry, scaly skin on the legs.

Callouses and Brittle Nails

Warm 250 ml (1 cup) olive or castor oil, add 125 ml (½ cup) sage leaves, and heat for 5 minutes. Stand, steep, cool and strain. Bottle. Rub frequently into callouses and nails, especially into cuticles.

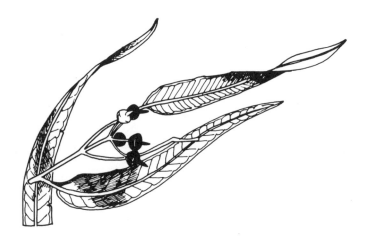

Chapped, Dry, Rough Skin Treatment

These dry areas can be rubbed with almond oil or sweet oil, in which scented geranium leaves have been steeped. Sweet oil is an excellent restorer, and with a few drops of eucalyptus or rosemary oil added to it, it is a most effective rub.

Brown Skin Spots

1 measure castor oil, eg 25 ml (2 tbsp)
1 measure wheatgerm oil
2 capsules vitamin E

Whirl in a blender, bottle, and apply frequently to the spots.

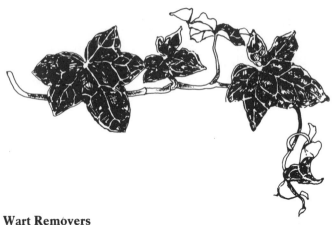

Wart Removers

The juice of a fig leaf, milkweed (*Asclepias*), ivy leaf, or purple tradescantia are all good wart removers. Alternatively make a poultice of a small pieces of the inside of a banana skin, or a piece of cotyledon leaf. Hold it in place over the wart with a strip of plaster. Replace daily with a fresh piece for a week to 10 days, or until the wart softens and falls off.

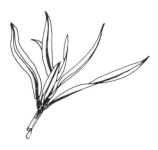

Chilblains

Make a strong infusion of calendula flowers (250 ml (1 cup) flowers to 250 ml (1 cup) boiling water). Soak the chilblains in this brew for 5-10 minutes or saturate a bandage and apply to the area. Dab on frequently.

An old-fashioned remedy is to rub ripe strawberries over the chilblain area daily throughout the season and the next winter the condition will ease. Make a strong tea of strawberry leaves and soak the chilblains in it daily when they trouble you.

Corn Remover

Soak several ivy leaves in enough apple cider vinegar to cover. Sprinkle with sea salt. Leave overnight or seal in a jar for a few days. Take out a leaf, apply it to the corn, and bind in place. The ivy leaves will gradually soften the corn until it can be lifted out. Massage the remaining scar with wheatgerm oil and vitamin E.

Foot Bath

This is a wonderful way of refreshing and reviving tired feet after a hard day.

Boil up a kettle of water, and pour it over any of the following herbs, 2 litres (8 cups) boiling water to 4 cups herbs: elder flowers and leaves, maidenhair fern, peppermint, pine-needles, rosemary, sage, yarrow, myrtle, mustard seeds, comfrey leaves, or castor oil leaves.

I first rub my feet with a little wheatgerm oil to which I have added a few drops of lavender oil. Then I immerse them in a basin of this brew, and soak for 10 minutes. Dry briskly and rub on a little soothing cream.

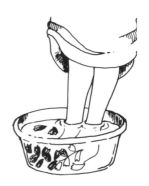

Quick Foot Refresher

Dip a few large castor oil leaves in hot water. Wrap them round your feet. Cover them with a warm towel, and sit back and relax for 15 minutes. In no time you'll be ready to go dancing.

Athlete's Foot Treatment

Athlete's foot is a most irritating fungal infection when the pH of the foot changes from acid to alkaline. To treat this condition effectively use apple cider vinegar in a foot bath three times a day. Wash the feet with soapwort, not soap, and allow the feet as much air as possible. Walk barefoot or wear open-toed sandals, but do be considerate when coming into contact with others as athlete's foot is highly infectious.

Herbal Bath for Athlete's Foot

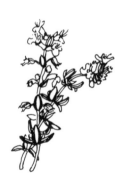

25 ml (2 tbsp) sage
25 ml (2 tbsp) calendula flowers
62,5 ml (5 tbsp) apple cider vinegar
25 ml (2 tbsp) thyme
1–2 litres (4–8 cups) water

Boil up the herbs in the water in a covered pot for 15 minutes. Cool. Strain. Add the vinegar. Save the strained herbs to rub between the toes. Immerse the feet in the 'tea' and sit down for half an hour and relax. Dry the feet meticulously. Do this daily until the condition clears.

Foot Massage

Having a foot massage is pure heaven and this oil is wonderfully soothing and relaxing after a hard day.

125 ml (1/2 cup) comfrey leaves
125 ml (1/2 cup) elder flowers
125 ml (1/2 cup) almond oil
10 ml (2 tsp) borax
10 ml (2 tsp) honey
250 ml (1 cup) sweet oil

Blend all the ingredients in a liquidiser. Rub into the feet, then wash off with warm water. Store excess in the refrigerator. This mixture is also excellent for aching legs and it does wonders for the skin.

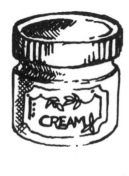

NAIL CARE

Cuticle Softener

25 ml (2 tbsp) fresh pineapple juice
25 ml (2 tbsp) pawpaw
1 egg yolk
5 ml (1 tsp) apple cider vinegar

Mash the pawpaw and mix into pineapple juice. Beat in the egg yolk. Add the cider vinegar and pour into a small bowl. Soak nails in the mixture for half an hour, massaging every now and then. Both pineapple and pawpaw contain an enzyme which softens protein tissue.

Cream for Damaged Nails

125 ml (¹/₂ cup) honey
1 egg yolk
125 ml (¹/₂ cup) avocado oil or castor oil
2 ml (¹/₂ tsp) sea salt

Beat ingredients together and keep in a screw-top jar in the refrigerator. Rub a little into the nails daily, leaving on for half an hour.

Nail Strengtheners

Warm up a little medicinal olive oil in a double boiler with a sprig or two of sage. Rub into the nails and cuticles.

Rub cider vinegar into the nails daily.

Rub lemon peel into the nails daily.

Rub glycerine into the nails daily.

Include calcium-rich foods in your diet and drink plenty of milk, yoghurt and buttermilk. Put herb teas, fresh fruit and fresh salads on your daily menu.

Make a lotion of 12,5 ml (1 tbsp) rosewater, 12,5 ml (1 tbsp) lemon juice, 12,5 ml (1 tbsp) glycerine, and 37,5 ml (3 tbsp) vodka. Pour into a bottle. Shake ingredients together and rub into nails and cuticles daily.

ORAL CARE

Natural Mouth Cleansers

Several herbs freshen and cleanse the mouth and teeth very effectively.

Fresh sage leaves rubbed over gums or chewed are very refreshing and cleanse the breath too.

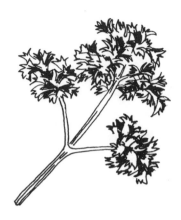

Fresh strawberries, both the cultivated type and the little bright wild strawberry, will clean stains and remove tartar from the teeth, as well as whiten them and invigorate the gums. Rub over teeth and gums every now and then.

Parsley chewed daily tightens loose teeth and keeps the gums healthy.

Massage a sliver of lemon peel into the gums to strengthen them and clear infections.

To ease toothache, chew a couple of cloves.

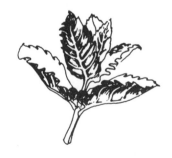

Mint Breath Fresheners

25 ml (2 tbsp) chopped mint
5 ml (1 tsp) finely crushed cloves
little egg white

Mix mint and cloves with a little egg white. Roll into tiny balls. Store until dry. Chew a mint freshener every now and then.

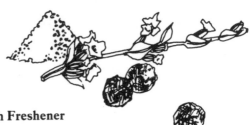

Lavender Breath Freshener

12,5 ml (1 tbsp) lavender flowers
25 ml (2 tbsp) icing sugar
2–3 drops lavender oil
1 egg white, whisked

Mix ingredients well, make into little balls, and leave to dry until firm. Chew when needed.

Chapped Lip Salve

Cold weather, wind-burn or sunburn often leave lips very sore and rough. You can make a quick dressing by mixing 2 or 3 drops of oil of sage with 5 ml (1 tbsp) honey and applying it frequently with your fingertip. Alternatively, make your own salve:

12,5 ml (1 tbsp) beeswax
12,5 ml (1 tbsp) sweet almond oil or medicinal olive oil
12,5 ml (1 tbsp) wheatgerm oil
3 drops oil of rosemary or lavender

Melt all ingredients in the top of a double boiler, stirring thoroughly. Cool, pour into a jar and keep covered. Smear a little every now and then onto sore lips.

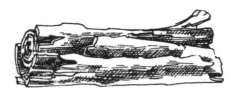

Spicy Mouthwash

25 ml (2 tbsp) crushed cloves
25 ml (2 tbsp) crushed nutmeg
12,5 ml (1 tbsp) crushed cinnamon
12,5 ml (1 tbsp) caraway seeds
few drops lavender oil
12,5 ml (1 tbsp) crushed allspice berries
500 ml (2 cups) sherry

Grind all the ingredients together and add to the sherry. Bottle and stand for 4 days, shaking up daily. This is a concentrated mouthwash and very cleansing, but it needs to be diluted. Use a few drops in a glass of water.

EYE CARE

Sparkling clear eyes are your most beautiful asset. To keep them this way mild herb infusions are very effective. To soothe tired eyes, make a mild tea, using 125 ml (½ cup) herb to 500 ml (2 cups) boiling water of cornflowers, calendula flowers, parsley, chamomile or fennel. A slice of cucumber placed over each eyelid is also excellent. Lie down and relax for 10 minutes.

Ordinary cold tea also makes a good eye lotion and tea bags soaked in warm tea, wrung out and applied to the eyelids will reduce puffiness. Another way to reduce puffiness is to grate a raw potato and put a teaspoon or two on a small square of lint. Cover the eyes and relax for 10–20 minutes. Splash with cold water.

HERB DEODORANTS

Several herbs are helpful in combating body odour. Those most often used through the centuries are sage, rosemary, leaves of chrysanthemum, lovage, celery and parsley. All can be made into a tea which is then used as a wash. Celery,

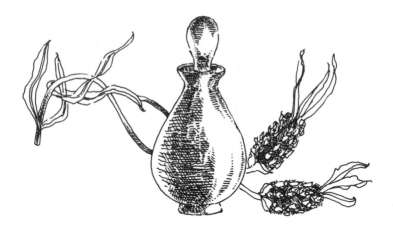

parsley, sage, rosemary and lovage should also be included frequently in the diet.

Lavender oil is also an excellent deodoriser and a strong lavender tea, 250 ml (1 cup) herb to 250 ml (1 cup) boiling water, can be used as a wash, adding a few drops of the oil before using.

Anti-perspirant Drink

This is an old-fashioned drink which is well worth trying.

rind of 1 lemon
250 ml (1 cup) milk
3 drops oil of camphor

Gently warm the milk and soak the lemon rind in it for 10 minutes. Add the oil of camphor. Drink the milk just before going to bed.

Apple cider vinegar makes an excellent wash for dispelling body odour and keeping the acid mantle of the skin.

Dilute 12,5 ml (1 tbsp) apple cider vinegar in 250 ml (1 cup) water and use frequently as a wash. Don't be put off by the smell of the vinegar; it evaporates in about 10 minutes.

Try to include chlorophyll-rich foods in your diet. The green of the vegetables is a natural deodoriser and green salads will not only keep your skin fresh but keep it clear of impurities.

HERBAL DOUCHES

Douching sensibly and in moderation is an excellent way to keep the vagina healthy and free from smell.

NB Pregnant women should never douche.

Cleansing Douche

½ litre (2 cups) boiling water
12,5 ml (1 tbsp) lavender leaves
12,5 ml (1 tbsp) apple cider vinegar
12,5 ml (1 tbsp) sage

Pour the boiling water over the herbs. Stand and steep. Allow to cool until warm. Strain. Add the vinegar and use as a douche.

Menstrual Disorder Douche

25 ml (2 tbsp) yarrow leaves and flowers
½ litre (2 cups) boiling water
25 ml (2 tbsp) mint

Pour boiling water over the herbs. Stand and steep. Strain when lukewarm. This douche will help to ease menstrual pain and stem a heavy flow.

Aphrodisiac Douche

25 ml (2 tbsp) scented geranium leaves
25 ml (2 tbsp) violet flowers
½ litre (2 cups) boiling water
25 ml (2 tbsp) myrtle

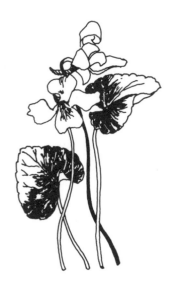

Pour boiling water over the herbs. Stand and steep. Strain when lukewarm. Use as a douche. These three beautifully fragrant herbs are believed to arouse passion – hence the name!

SUNBURN

Sunburn is a very common complaint throughout long, hot summers and one we should take pains to avoid, for it has an ageing and drying effect on the skin.

Sun Protection Oil

This protecting oil should be applied before going out into the sun. The sesame oil blots out the harmful ultra-violet rays.

25 ml (2 tbsp) sesame oil
25 ml (2 tbsp) lanolin
75 ml (6 tbsp) dandelion tea or elder flower tea

Melt lanolin and oil in a double boiler. Slowly add the warm herb infusion. Mix well. Bottle and apply liberally to the skin.

Citrus Sun Oil

25 ml (2 tbsp) sesame oil
25 ml (2 tbsp) grated lemon peel
25 ml (2 tbsp) lanolin
50 ml (4 tbsp) strong tea

Melt lanolin and sesame oil in a double boiler. Add the lemon peel. Simmer on a low heat for half an hour. Add tea, and strain. Apply to the skin frequently when out in the sun.

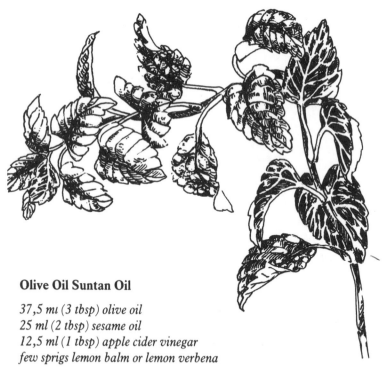

Olive Oil Suntan Oil

37,5 ml (3 tbsp) olive oil
25 ml (2 tbsp) sesame oil
12,5 ml (1 tbsp) apple cider vinegar
few sprigs lemon balm or lemon verbena

Mix all ingredients together, pour into a bottle, and shake frequently. Apply before going out in the sun.

Soothing Cream for Sunburn

37,5 ml (3 tbsp) anhydrous lanolin
12,5 ml (1 tbsp) wheatgerm oil
37,5 ml (3 tbsp) strong comfrey tea, using root and leaf, 250 ml
* (1 cup) herb to 250 ml (1 cup) boiling water*
37,5 ml (3 tbsp) apple cider vinegar

Blend all ingredients in a blender. Bottle and apply to painful areas.

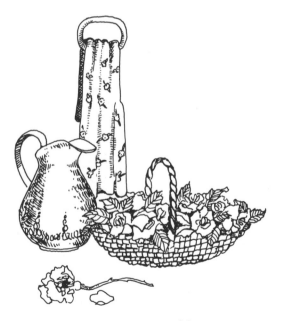

Hair Care

A head of beautifully clean, bouncy, shiny hair is indeed an enviable asset. Once again, in order to achieve those smooth, shiny locks, you need to eat foods that are fresh and healthy – plenty of fruit, vegetables and salads. Drink lots of water and make sure that you get enough sleep – eight hours each night will do wonders for your hair. Regular shampooing, conditioning and brushing will further serve to beautify it and is well worth the effort. Old-fashioned beauty tips like adding egg to shampoo as a protein conditioner for dry hair, and lemon juice in tepid water as a final rinse for oily hair, still hold good. And rosemary, nettle or yarrow tea rubbed into the scalp will stimulate hair growth.

The vast array of shampoos, conditioners and setting lotions available today can be confusing. The general trend, however, is to the natural shampoos that are now on the market. Take a close look at the ingredients to find a product which is suitable for your particular hair type. To give the shampoo that extra something add a herb tea or infusion, eg chamomile, rosemary or nettle.

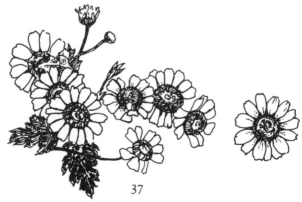

For fair hair, make a strong chamomile tea (1 cup flowers to 500 ml (2 cups) boiling water). Allow to stand and steep, then strain and add to the shampoo, in equal quantities of tea and shampoo. Shake well and shampoo in the normal way. Chamomile is a softener and brings out the highlights in fair hair. For dark hair, add rosemary or sage tea to shampoo; these are both revitalising herbs. For normal or oily hair, add some verbascum flower or nettle tea, or a beaten egg white. For dry, brittle hair, add a beaten egg yolk.

Herbal Shampoo

250 ml (1 cup) nettles, yarrow or rosemary
500 ml (2 cups) boiling water

Pour boiling water over the herbs. Stand and allow to steep for 20 minutes, then strain. Pour the tea into an enamel saucepan and shave into it 1 cup of a good, pure soap (I use a baby soap or goatmilk soap). Heat the mixture, stirring constantly until the soap is melted. Then set aside to cool. When it is lukewarm, add a few drops of essential oil, eg rose, jasmine, honeysuckle, lavender etc (my favourite is rosemary). Pour into a bottle and use as a shampoo. Shake up just before using. This shampoo will keep for about a month.

Herbal Shampoo for Oily Hair

250 ml (1 cup) yarrow
500 ml (2 cups) boiling water
25 ml (2 tbsp) apple cider vinegar

Pour boiling water over the yarrow. Add cider vinegar. Stand and allow to steep for 20 minutes, then strain. Pour the tea into an enamel saucepan and shave into it 1 cup of a good, pure soap (a baby soap or goatmilk soap). Heat the mixture, stirring constantly until the soap has melted. Set aside to cool. When it is lukewarm, add a few drops of essential oil, eg rose, jasmine, honeysuckle, lavender, rosemary. Pour into a bottle and use as a shampoo. Shake up just before using.

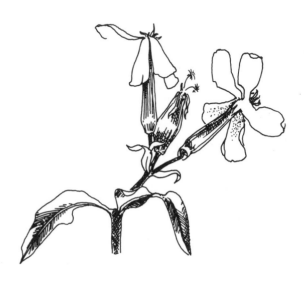

Soapwort Shampoo

Shampoo your hair once with an ordinary shampoo. Then shampoo and soak your hair in soapwort shampoo. This is made by boiling up a potful of soapwort leaves, flowers, roots and stems in just enough water to cover them. Boil for 20 minutes, keeping the pot covered. (Use an enamel or stainless steel pot.) Remove from the heat, stand until cool, and strain before using. Soak the hair in it as long as possible. Rinse with rosemary water. This is especially effective for dry, over-permed, over-dyed or heat-damaged hair. It is also good for dry, unmanageable hair after an anaesthetic or a long illness.

Herbal Rinse to Stimulate Growth

250 ml (1 cup) nettles
125 ml (½ cup) rosemary
125 ml (½ cup) southernwood
125 ml (½ cup) watercress
125 ml (½ cup) yarrow
1 litre (4 cups) water (rainwater if possible)
25 ml (2 tbsp) cider vinegar

Boil up the herbs in the water for 5 minutes, then set aside to cool. Strain. Add the cider vinegar. Use this rinse on your hair after shampooing. Massage well into the scalp.

Treatment for Damaged Hair

This is a special monthly treatment that works wonders on hair which has lost its lustre, or is brittle and falling out. It is excellent, too, for over-bleached and dyed hair.

Brush clean hair vigorously, bending forward from the waist so that the head falls forward. Choose an unsaturated oil such as wheatgerm, maize, sunflower or almond oil, and heat 1 cup of oil until just hot enough so as not to be uncomfortable. Add 6 drops of rosemary or lavender oil. Wet hair well, then towel dry. Saturate a pad of cotton-wool in the oil and apply to the scalp, sectioning the hair out of the way until it has all been covered. Massage the oil in deeply. Wring out a hand towel in hot herb water – as hot as you can bear. Pour 3 litres (12 cups) boiling water over 500 ml (2 cups) rosemary or nettles. Let it cool a little before straining. Wrap the hot towel turban-like over the head. Cover with a plastic shower cap.

As soon as the scalp feels cool, repeat the hot, wet towel procedure – or sit under a hot lamp or hair dryer to maintain the heat. Try to keep the treatment going for at least an hour. Wash out with a good shampoo. You will probably need 2 or 3 shampoos to get the oil out completely. Make a herbal brew, adding a dash of apple cider vinegar, as the final rinse. Rosemary makes a good brew – 500 ml (2 cups) rosemary in 4–5 cups boiling water. Stand until just pleasantly warm enough to use.

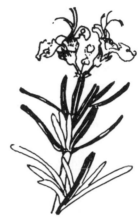

Herbal Conditioner for Oily Hair

Don't think oily hair needs no conditioning; it needs it as much as dry hair, and a monthly treatment will ensure that your hair keeps its bounce and lustre.

75 ml (6 tbsp) rum
75 ml (6 tbsp) strong yarrow tea
3 egg yolks, well beaten

Liquidise all ingredients together. Wet the hair well. Section the hair and apply this mixture to each section, using cotton-wool pads. Rub into the scalp and hair. Meanwhile have a strong infusion of yarrow and rosemary tea warming on the stove. Dip a small towel into it and wring it out, as hot as you can bear. Wrap it around your head. Cover with a shower-cap to keep the heat in. Have another hot towel ready to replace the first one as it cools, the aim being to keep the hair warm to absorb the conditioner. Try to keep the treatment going for an hour. Finally, wash out with a good shampoo and rinse with yarrow tea.

Setting Lotions

For oily hair

250 ml (1 cup) skimmed milk with 10 ml (2 tsp) sea salt
  dissolved in it

beer

strong herb infusion, eg yarrow, lavender, rosemary, 250 ml
  (1 cup) herb to 500 ml (2 cups) boiling water

For dry hair

lemon juice
strong maidenhair fern tea, 1 cup fern, well pressed down, to
  250 ml (1 cup) boiling water. Stand for 10 minutes. Strain.

Setting lotion

1 egg white and 10 ml (2 tsp) gelatine, whisked in 250 ml
  (1 cup) boiling water, then combed into the hair

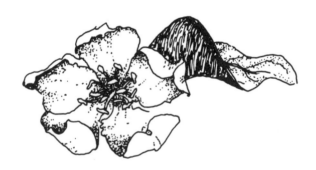

Herbal Treatment for Falling Hair

Boil up equal quantities herb and rainwater for 5 minutes. Use
any of the following, or combinations thereof: globe artichoke
leaves, lavender leaves and flowers, maidenhair fern, calendula

flowers and a few leaves, nasturtium flowers and a few leaves, nettle, quince peels, cores, leaves or blossom, rosemary, southernwood, thyme, vine leaves, watercress, and willow leaves. Allow to cool, then strain. To every litre (4 cups) herbal infusion, add 120 ml (½ cup) vodka. Dab this mixture liberally into the roots of the hair every day, but do not rub too strongly as this will encourage the hair to fall out. The mixture will last about a month; the vodka acts as a preservative.

To Thicken Hair and Encourage Growth

This is an old-fashioned mixture which should be applied once a month.

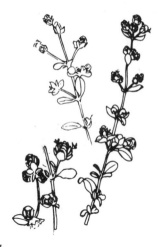

250 ml (1 cup) honey
250 ml (1 cup) almond oil
250 ml (1 cup) strong marjoram tea for dark hair or 250 ml (1 cup) strong chamomile tea for fair hair

Put ingredients through a liquidiser, then rub the mixture into the scalp. Cover with a plastic shower-cap and leave on for half an hour. Shampoo in the normal way. Use a rosemary or basil rinse to cleanse. Keep any excess in the refrigerator for the next time.

Natural Treatment for Damaged Hair

Eggs probably make the best protein treatment for brittle hair. This amazing treatment should be applied once a week to put strength and lustre back into damaged hair. Once your hair is looking good again, use the treatment monthly to keep it that way.

37,5 ml (3 tbsp) castor oil
37,5 ml (3 tbsp) lanolin
25 ml (2 tbsp) medicinal olive oil
50 ml (4 tbsp) glycerine
12,5 ml (1 tbsp) shampoo
310 ml (1¼ cups) warm water
2 eggs
2 extra egg yolks
10 ml (2 tsp) apple cider vinegar
few drops lavender oil

In the top of a double boiler melt and blend castor oil, lanolin and olive oil. Remove from heat and stand for 5 minutes. Using an electric mixer on a low speed, or an egg beater, slowly whisk in glycerine, shampoo and water. As it thickens whisk in the egg yolks, cider vinegar and the essential oil. Pour into a screw-top jar and refrigerate (be sure to label it or someone may mistake it for mayonnaise!). The next day add 2 eggs, beaten at high speed, and apply to newly shampooed hair. Cover with a shower-cap for at least one hour, then shampoo out. Finish up with a herbal rinse.

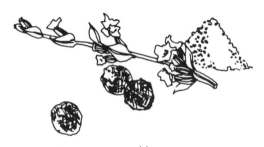

Quick Protein Conditioner

This is an excellent weekly conditioner, quick and easy to make.

2 eggs
12,5 ml (1 tbsp) castor oil
12,5 ml (1 tbsp) wheatgerm oil
12,5 ml (1 tbsp) glycerine
10 ml (2 tsp) apple cider vinegar

Beat all ingredients together briskly. Apply to hair after the initial shampoo. Cover with a shower-cap for 15–20 minutes (half an hour, if you have the time, is ideal). Shampoo out and use a herbal tea as a final rinse.

Restoring Lustre to Dull Hair

Dry hair

250 ml (1 cup) strong rosemary tea, 250 ml (1 cup) herb to 250 ml
  (1 cup) boiling water
12,5 ml (1 tbsp) sweet almond oil
few drops rosemary or lavender oil

Use as a setting lotion or brush a little into the hair after shampooing.

Oily hair

2 eggs
250 ml (1 cup) rum
250 ml (1 cup) freshly made rosewater (boil up 500 ml (2 cups)
  rose petals in 375 ml (1½ cups) water for 5 minutes.
  Stand, cool, strain)

Whisk eggs and rum into rosewater and massage through the hair. Leave on for 15 minutes. Rinse with a herbal rinse.

Dandruff

A dry, flaky scalp indicates a sloughing off of matured skin cells and a few flakes is quite normal. It is only when this becomes excessive that it has to be considered a problem. There are two types of dandruff, one oily and one dry. Oily dandruff is usually found amongst adolescents and adults with an excessively oily scalp. Dermatologists often recommend cutting out oily foods in the diet, fatty, fried food, chocolate, butter and iodised salt. There are several ways of treating dandruff and once again there is no better way to start than to include salads and fruit and lots of fresh water in the diet. Correct eating goes a long way to improving the condition. Other methods worth trying are as follows:

Brushing: Vigorous daily brushing helps increase the circulation of blood to the scalp.

Vinegars: One of the quickest ways to remove dandruff is to massage herbal vinegars into the scalp; the irritating itch will disappear at the same time. Make herbal vinegars – rosemary, nettle, yarrow, bay, basil, sage, marjoram etc (see Bathtime Herbs), or use apple cider vinegar. Rub into the scalp daily.

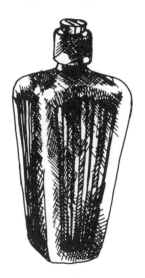

Oils: Massage warm oil into the hair and scalp once or twice a week. Use castor oil, sweet oil, wheatgerm oil or maize oil. After massaging the oil well in, put on a plastic shower-cap, and keep covered with a towel for half an hour. Shampoo with a mild shampoo and rinse with a herbal vinegar or infusion.

Lemon juice: Massage freshly squeezed lemon juice into the scalp after shampooing. Rinse out with rosemary tea.

Rosemary and nettle paste: Pour 250 ml (1 cup) boiling water over 250 ml (1 cup) nettle leaves. Liquidise. Add 500 ml (2 cups) finely minced rosemary and 37,5 ml (3 tbsp) borax. Rub this paste into the scalp just after shampooing. Rinse out with a herbal infusion.

Astringent hair rinse: This rinse is good for all hair types. It closes the pores and removes dandruff. Take 250 ml (1 cup) each: comfrey leaves, scented geranium leaves and sweet basil leaves. Simmer in a litre (4 cups) water. Cool and strain. Add 125 ml (½ cup) apple cider vinegar. Massage into the scalp.

Natural Hair Colouring

There are several natural hair colourings that will gently tint the hair. They are infinitely preferable to harsh commercial dyes which can damage the delicate hair shafts.

Reddish colouring

Boil up equal quantities of radish leaves and radishes with privet or myrtle leaves, in enough water to cover them. Use as a wash and a rinse.

Brown colouring

Make a strong sage tea (250 ml (1 cup) herb to 500 ml (2 cups) boiling water) and use as a rinse.

Crush 20 green walnuts, shells, leaves and husks. Cover with water, add 12,5 ml (1 tbsp) salt, and a few more leaves. Stand overnight. Strain. Rub into the hair.

Use ivy berries to make a strong tea, and use as a rinse.

Raspberry leaves and red poppies can also be made into a strong tea (250 ml (1 cup) herb to 500 ml (2 cups) boiling water) and used as a rinse.

To blacken hair and darken grey hair

Artichoke leaves (globe artichoke), marjoram and elderberries are all effective hair darkeners. Boil up any one of them in enough rainwater to cover. Stand overnight. Strain, and use as a rinse.

Arab remedy for darkening grey hair

Thinly peel 6 green oranges. Steep the peel in maize oil or sunflower oil, just enough to cover the peels. Store for 3 months. Strain and comb the oil through the hair. Cover with a shower-cap and leave on for half an hour. Shampoo in the normal way. Use this once a week and you'll soon notice a rich darkening of grey hair.

Fair hair

To lighten hair make a strong herbal tea, using chamomile flowers, verbascum flowers, privet or myrtle flowers, or rhubarb root. Use as a rinse.

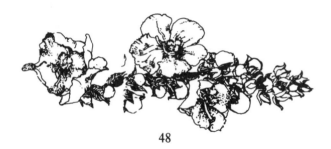

Bathtime Herbs

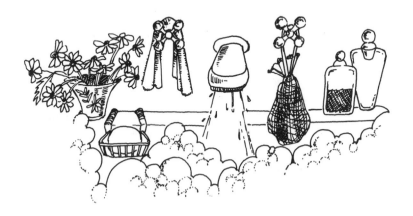

I don't know anyone who doesn't enjoy a luxurious warm bath, as a relaxing end to a long day or as a refreshing early start before a day's work. The simplest, most inexpensive and pleasurable way of using herbs, whether to soften or invigorate and tone the skin, or to relax, soothe and scent the body, is by adding them to the bathwater.

There are various ways of doing this. Try tying a bunch of herbs in a square of muslin or net, or in the foot of an old stocking, and suspending it under the hot water tap. Rub the bag briskly over your body like a sponge, and then lie back and relax in the herb-scented water.

Another method is to make a strong infusion of whatever herb you prefer. Pour over enough boiling water to cover a big bowl of fresh herbs, well pressed down. Stand for 15 minutes, strain and pour the liquid into the bathwater.

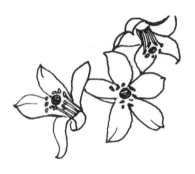

Herbs suitable for using in the bath are: the mints, lemon verbena, lemon balm (melissa), lavender, sage, rosemary, elder flowers and leaves, soapwort leaves, flowers, roots and stems, calendula, scented geranium, bergamot, lemon peel, orange blossom, jasmine flowers, comfrey and southernwood.

BATH VINEGARS

These are an easy way of making a bath fragrant and softening the water, leaving your skin soft and fresh. Used regularly in winter in dry climates, bath vinegars will keep your skin from drying and flaking. All you need is a little time to get the vinegars smelling rich and fragrant.

I use a 5-litre bottle of white vinegar and fill it with a favourite herb. (Remove a cup or two and fill another, smaller bottle to keep in the bathroom cupboard.) Steep the herb in the vinegar. Stand in the sun for about 3 weeks, replacing the herbs with fresh ones every 5 or 6 days. Strain through muslin and re-bottle, placing a sprig of fresh herb in each bottle for identification. Use a dash or two in the bath, for rinsing the hair, or for dabbing onto tired, aching feet.

Any fragrant herb will do, eg lavender, rosemary, scented geranium, lemon verbena, red rose petals, or orange blossom. Try combining herbs and flowers. A lovely spring bath vinegar can be made using jasmine flowers with mint, or orange blossom and lemon verbena. You will derive much pleasure from experimenting. Bath vinegars also make lovely gifts.

Apple Cider Vinegar Invigorator

1 bottle apple cider vinegar
1 piece fresh root ginger, about 4 cm long
2–4 sprigs rosemary
2–6 sprigs sage

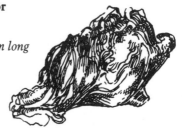

Press the herbs into the vinegar. Stand in the sun for 3 weeks. Change the herbs once each week. Strain and re-bottle. Use a little in the bath, or to soothe tired muscles, dabbing on with cotton-wool.

HERBAL BATH OILS

Although there is a huge variety of commercial bath oils, I find it far more rewarding and satisfying to make my own out of pure, natural ingredients. Most oils merely float on the surface of the water, but you can buy a soluble bath oil, unscented and uncoloured, from chemists which dissolves in the water and is absorbed by the skin. Almond oil, maize oil, sunflower oil, sweet oil, or avocado oil are also suitable.

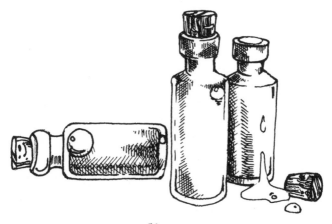

Herbal bath oils are all made in the same way. Choose a favourite herb, eg rosemary, and push several sprigs or leaves into a bottle of oil. Stand out of direct sunlight for 3 weeks. Replace the herb each week with fresh sprigs. Then strain and add a few drops of essential oil (if you have used rosemary, then add rosemary essential oil as a fragrance). If you like you can add a little wheatgerm oil which has the added advantage of nourishing the skin and preserving the oil. Use sparingly in the bath.

Bubble Bath Oil

This is a nourishing and softening oil and children love it.

250 ml (1 cup) good quality soap, grated
1 litre (4 cups) boiling water, into which 6 sprigs rosemary or
*   lavender, approx 20 cm long, have been steeped for 15 minutes*
25 ml (2 tbsp) witch-hazel
50 ml (4 tbsp) glycerine
12,5 ml (1 tbsp) wheatgerm oil
few drops lavender oil

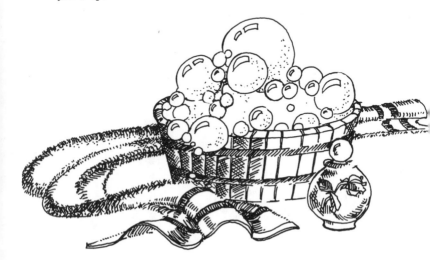

Dissolve the soap in the herb 'tea'. Whisk glycerine, wheat-germ, essential oil and witch-hazel, then pour into a liquidiser with the soap mixture. Liquidise for 5 minutes, then pour into a screw-top bottle and add 25 ml (2 tbsp) water from the hot tap. Pour a few drops into the bathwater and lie back and relax.

Sweet Oil Skin Softener

500 ml (2 cups) sweet oil
250 ml (1 cup) calendula flowers
few drops honeysuckle essential oil

Steep flowers in the sweet oil in a screw-top bottle, adding a few drops honeysuckle essential oil. Stand for 2 weeks, shaking every now and then. Use a few drops in the bath or as a rub into dry skin. If you strain the flowers out after 2 weeks the oil will keep indefinitely.

Soothing Almond Bath Oil

250 ml (1 cup) sunflower oil
500 ml (2 cups) almond oil
250 ml (1 cup) scented geranium leaves
125 ml (1/2 cup) wheatgerm oil
few drops scented geranium oil

Combine the almond, sunflower and wheatgerm oils. Steep the scented geranium leaves in the oil for 2–3 weeks. Twice or 3 times during that time, strain out the geranium leaves and pack with fresh ones (before throwing away the used scented leaves, I toss them into my bath to have the benefit of every tiny drop of oil! Take care that they don't block the drain.) Strain out the leaves, add the essential oil, shake well in a screw-top bottle and add a teaspoon or two to the bathwater.

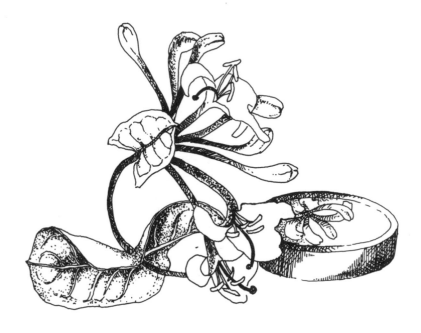

HERBAL SOAPS

Making soap from scratch is a complicated and time-consuming business, and for most people, whose lives are full and busy, far too involved and difficult – even dangerous if you are not an expert, as an alkaline can burn the skin as badly as acid. So leave soap-making to the experts and rather choose a plain soap which suits your skin and grate it. You can then add herbs, oatmeal, honey etc, using the recipes below as a guide. They are quick and easy to make and have been tested and proved suitable for most skin types. Experiment on your own (always test with care) for you will get infinite satisfaction and pleasure out of making your own beauty preparations.

Rich Moisturising Soap

500 ml (2 cups) grated plain soap
25 ml (2 tbsp) lanolin
25 ml (2 tbsp) honey
12,5 ml (1 tbsp) rosewater
5 ml (1 tsp) essential oil of rose or rose geranium

Place the grated soap in the top of a double boiler and simmer gently (I find if the water boils too vigorously, I have a hard time beating and blending). As it starts to melt add the honey and lanolin. Stir gently all the time until it is blended, then add the essential oil and mix well. Line a soap dish or small bowl with clingwrap or thin tinfoil (to prevent sticking) and pour in the soap mixture. When the soap has solidified remove it from the container and keep it in an airy place for about 10 days to allow it to mature. Then take a bath with it and enjoy it!

Honey and Lemon Dry Skin Soap

This is a nourishing soap for dry skin, and is particularly good for legs and feet.

500 ml (2 cups) grated plain soap
125 ml (½ cup) honey
25 ml (2 tbsp) finely grated lemon skin or rind
12,5 ml (1 tbsp) lemon juice
5 ml (1 tsp) oil of lemon

Use the same method as for the Rich Moisturising Soap.

Soft Herb Soap

This is a jelly-like soap that should be kept in a jar beside the wash basin. I use it for washing my hands frequently and, as a potter, when my hands get very rough and sore it has been my salvation many a time.

250 ml (1 cup) borax
500 ml (2 cups) grated plain soap
25 ml (2 tbsp) rosemary
25 ml (2 tbsp) lemon thyme
25 ml (2 tbsp) sage
25 ml (2 tbsp) lemon verbena
250 ml (1 cup) comfrey leaves, chopped
enough water to cover the herbs, approx 375–500 ml (1½–2 cups)
5 ml (1 tsp) rosemary oil

Place the herbs in a stainless steel pot (never use aluminium) and bring to the boil with the lid on. Remove from the stove and stand until cool. Strain. Grate the soap and place it in the top of a double boiler over gently simmering water.

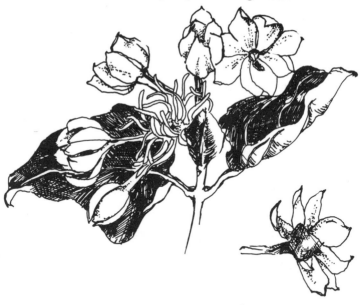

Dissolve the borax in the herbal infusion and add to the soap, a little at a time. Stir gently until the soap has melted. Add a little essential oil, blend well, and pour into a screw-top jar.

As this soap contains so many herbs, it will not keep indefinitely but if it is kept well closed, it will keep a little longer. It is so easy to make, however, that you should use it lavishly and make fresh batches frequently.

I often change the herbs during the year as the mood takes me and the experiments are great fun. Try the following: elder flowers and leaves, lavender flowers and leaves, scented geranium leaves, myrtle flowers and leaves, sour fig leaves, chamomile flowers and leaves, bergamot flowers and leaves, marjoram flowers and leaves, lemon skin and leaves, orange blossom, calendula flowers, jasmine flowers, borage flowers and leaves, hypericum flowers.

Comfrey, incidentally, is very soothing so always try to include it in your ingredients. In fact, this list includes many healing, soothing herbs, and you will have to test your own to find your favourites.

Herb and Oatmeal Soap

This soap is the only one I make from caustic soda.

NB Do not underestimate caustic soda — it is a hazardous chemical that needs very careful handling. Wear eye protection, long sleeves and rubber gloves. Caustic soda flakes are safer to handle than granules or sticks; use outdoors and take great care not to breathe the dust. Do not lean over the bowl and inhale. Do not use containers of aluminium or zinc, as caustic soda attacks these metals. When preparing a solution, add the caustic soda slowly and carefully to the water — never the other way round, because much heat is generated as it dissolves. Should a drop fall on your skin, wash off immediately with lots of cold water.

50 g (2 oz) fresh herb, eg rosemary, lemon verbena, comfrey, elder,
  lavender, scented geranium, finely minced
150 ml (¼ pt) boiling water
15 ml (3 tsp) caustic soda
300 ml (½ pt) almond oil
100 g (4 oz) coconut oil
12,5 ml (1 tbsp) glycerine
25 ml (2 tbsp) fine oatmeal
10 ml (2 tbsp) essential oil, eg rosemary, lemon verbena etc

Line 2 or 3 small soap dishes or bowls with clingwrap, thin tinfoil, waxed paper or (my favourite) a piece of fine material wrung out in water.

Pour the boiling water over the chopped herb and infuse for 20–30 minutes. Strain into a glass or china bowl, then very carefully stir in the caustic soda (I sprinkle in a little at a time). Leave until lukewarm. Put the oils and the glycerine into an enamel or stainless steel pot and gently warm to dissolve. Then very carefully pour the oil and glycerine mixture into the herb and caustic soda mixture and stir with a wooden spoon until it thickens (about 15–20 minutes). If you have an electric beater, put it on to the lowest speed. The stirring/beating is essential as there is a chemical reaction between the ingredients which makes the 'soapiness'.

Gradually stir in the oatmeal, herb and the essential oil. Pour into the lined and prepared moulds, cover with a clean cloth and allow to set for 2–3 days.

When the soap is set take it out of the mould, wrap it in fresh wax paper and leave to mature in a cool, dry cupboard for 2–3 weeks.

WASH BALLS

This covers anything from a handful of fresh herbs tied up in muslin or net, a lump of shaved soap mixed into herbs and spices, to a bath bag of herbs and soap. Here are a few ideas, all of which are a delight to use:

Lavender Wash Balls

500 ml (2 cups) dried lavender leaves and flowers
750 ml (3 cups) grated lavender soap
25–75 ml (2–6 tbsp) fine oatmeal
12,5 ml (1 tbsp) lavender essential oil
250 ml (1 cup) boiling water

Place the soap and the water into the top of a double boiler and melt gently until soft. Stir in the herbs and the oatmeal. Blend well, then add the essential oil.

Take tablespoons and place in heaps on greased paper. Allow to harden for about a week. Tie the washballs up in squares of nylon net and use as a sponge. Place them in a bath glove, or use as a soap.

SOAP SUBSTITUTES

Soapwort

Many people are allergic to soap. If that is your problem try making a strong brew of saponin-containing soapwort (*Saponaria officinalis*) which is both mild and at the same time cleansing.

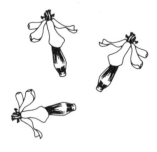

This common garden plant, known as 'Bouncing Bet', is actually a pest in the garden, as it spreads everywhere and you can never get rid of it. Its wonderful healing, cleansing and revitalising properties, however, make up for its nuisance value. Line the garden bed with thick pieces of plastic, to a depth of at least 50 cm, if you want to curb its encroaching habit.

Pick flowers, leaves, stems and roots, and fill a large enamel or stainless steel pot with them. Cover with water and bring to the boil. Boil for 15–20 minutes. Stand, steep, strain and use while still warm enough to be pleasant. Use as a soap for the face and body, and as a shampoo for brittle, dry, heat-damaged, dyed or tinted hair.

Almond Soap

This is a soothing soap substitute. Make a jarful at a time and use a knob for washing. It is particularly good for sunburnt skins. Smooth it on as you would a face pack and leave it for a few minutes before washing off with clear water.

25 ml (2 tbsp) almonds, finely ground
25 ml (2 tbsp) kaolin (fine white clay)
2–5 ml (½–1 tsp) borax
little almond oil

Mix all the ingredients together (the almond oil will bind them). Add a little rosewater if you like.

Herb Bath Bags

Fresh herbs such as scented geranium, lavender, myrtle, rosemary, sage, lemon verbena, or yarrow can be tied into a bundle in a square of net or pushed into an old stocking. Add a handful or two of large-flake oats and bran, and then use as a wash ball. The herbs will soften and cleanse the skin and the oats will soothe. This is a wonderful way of washing for those who are allergic to soap. Rub well into the skin and add a dash or two of herb vinegar to the bathwater to cleanse the skin of oiliness. Replace the herbs with fresh ones for each bath.

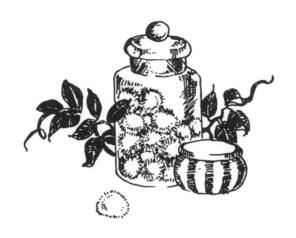

Herbs Used in Cosmetics

ALMOND (*Prunus communis, P. amygdalus, P. dulcis*)

Shelled almonds, ground into a meal and mixed with a herb infusion such as rosemary or sage, make an excellent mild bleaching face pack. They have a deep cleansing and toning effect.

Almond oil is non-drying and has superb emollient or softening properties; it also combines well with creams and, in lotions, with other ingredients. Can be used as a deep cleansing oil.

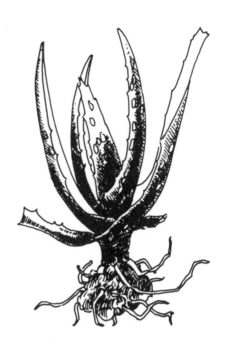

ALOE (*Aloe vera, A. arborescens*)

Most aloes can be used directly on the skin for burns. The juice can be included in various lotions and shampoos for its healing, soothing properties make it appealing. The juice of some aloes has a deep yellow colour which stains the skin, so use the clear fleshy leaves of *Aloe vera* to be on the safe side.

ANISE (*Pimpinella anisum*)

The seed of anise smells a little like licorice. A brew of crushed seeds and boiling water is used cosmetically in facial steams to open and medicate the pores. The same brew (250 ml (1 cup) seeds to 1–1½ litres (4–6 cups) boiling water) is excellent for rinsing the hair and enhancing its colour; at the same time it cleanses the pores of the scalp.

APPLE (*Malus sylvestris*)

Mashed fresh pulp of apple is astringent and toning on the skin and can be used in all sorts of masks, hand creams and scrubs. It is especially effective for sensitive or fair skins. A good soothing rub for rough skin, elbows, heels and knees, can be made by mixing fresh apple pulp with a little glycerine and rubbing into the area. Leave on for 10 minutes, then wash off. Apple pulp mixed with a little honey is a soothing balm for dry, sunburned, irritated skin.

Apple cider vinegar is a natural astringent. Dilute with water and use to tone and revitalise the skin. Used neat, it can be applied to spots and pimples to speed up the healing process. A dash added to a basin of water before washing your face is excellent, and it can also be used as a hair rinse or, neat, as a hair setting lotion.

APRICOT (*Prunus armeniaca*)

Fresh apricot pulp is marvellous for a sallow or oily skin. If apricots are not in season, you can use dried apricots soaked overnight and then boiled up to a pulp (I put in a sprig or two of sage when cooking the fruit). The pulp can then be mixed with yoghurt, oats, bran or buttermilk and used as a face pack. It deep cleanses and tones.

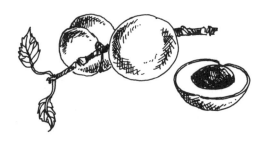

ASCLEPIAS (Milkweed, Swan plant)
(*Asclepias physocarpa*)

Our indigenous milkweed has the ability to open and cleanse pores if used as a cosmetic. The white milky juice is an effective treatment when applied directly to warts and pimples (remember to do a patch test first). Pour boiling water over the leaves and flowers to make a cleansing wash.

ASPARAGUS (*Asparagus officinalis*)

The new young spears of asparagus, boiled up in milk, act as a deep skin cleanser, and this is a particularly good treatment for acne and skin blemishes. Pat onto the skin with pads of cotton-wool and allow to dry. Wash off with tepid water.

AVOCADO (*Persea americana*)

Avocados contain potassium, sulphur and vitamins A, D and E, and these properties make them particularly useful for face and scalp packs. Pulp the flesh and use as a skin mask. The oil is obtainable from chemists and can be included in treatments, creams and lotions, or applied directly on its own to the skin.

BANANA (*Musa paradisiaca*)

Fresh ripe mashed banana makes an excellent mask for the face. It tightens and cleanses the pores, and invigorates and tones the skin. Leave on for 15 minutes. Wash off with tepid water.

BARLEY (*Hordeum* species)

Boil pearl barley – 250 ml (1 cup) barley grits to 1 litre (4 cups) boiling water – simmer slowly for 20–30 minutes and strain. Drink the barley water when cooled as a blood cleanser. A day on barley water cleanses the whole system – I find it more palatable with a little freshly squeezed lemon juice added. It is excellent for oily or problem skins and acne. Use the boiled barley grits as a scrub or pack on the face, neck, chest and back. Allow to dry, then wash off.

BASIL (*Ocimum basilicum*)

Basil leaves, boiled up in water (enough water to cover a layer of leaves and stalks), make an unsurpassed hair dressing or rinse. Basil assists hair growth, reduces tangles and snarls and it is a good scalp tonic. Rub well into the scalp after shampooing.

BAY LAUREL (*Laurus nobilis*)

Fresh bay leaves can be boiled up in water – 4 cups leaves to 6–8 cups water – and the resulting 'tea' can be rubbed into the scalp to stimulate hair growth. It can also be used as a splash-on after-shave lotion as it keeps the skin soft. It has a wonderful deep toning effect on the scalp and skin.

BEETROOT (*Beta vulgaris*)

Juice of fresh beetroot can be used as a lip colouring or rouge, and a tablespoon of mashed, cooked beetroot, mixed with 50 ml (4 tbsp) yoghurt, makes an excellent toning mask – leave for half an hour, then wash off with tepid water.

BERGAMOT (*Monarda didyma*)

A strong tea made of flowers and leaves – 500 ml (2 cups) herb to 1–1,5 litres (4–6 cups) boiling water – can be splashed onto the face as an astringent or used as a rinse for strengthening the hair. Taken as a tea, 60 ml (¼ cup) herb to 250 ml (1 cup) boiling water, it tones and stimulates the digestive organs. It is known as a cure-all health herb.

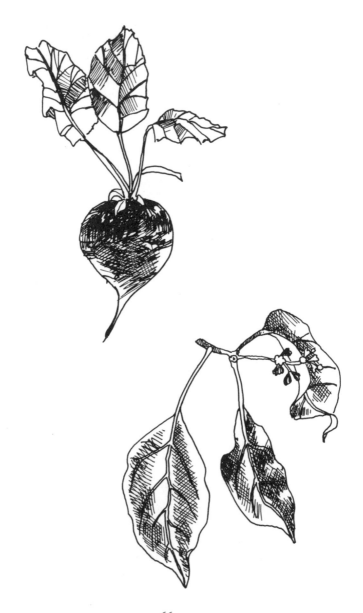

BORAGE (*Borago officinalis*)

Borage tea, 60 ml (¼ cup) herb to 250 ml (1 cup) boiling water, can be used as a wash for sores, scratches and spots. Taken internally, it is a wonderful cleanser and helps the body produce its own cortisone. It can be used as an eyewash and as a compress – dip cotton-wool into the tea and apply to the temples for stress and tension headaches.

CALENDULA (*Calendula officinalis*)

Flowers can be made into a strong tea (125 ml (½ cup) petals to 375 ml (1½ cups) boiling water) and used for skin blemishes, for baby's bath, as a wash for nappy rash, sunburn, and cradle cap. A poultice can be used for sores, bites and spots as it is both soothing and healing.

CAMPHOR (*Cinnamomum camphora*)

The slightly antiseptic camphor leaves can be made into a strong brew, used to rub directly onto stiff muscles or poured into the bath. Boil up 6–10 cups of leaves in enough water to cover them for 10 minutes.

CARAWAY (*Carum carvi*)

Leaves and seeds can be made into a poultice to reduce inflammation and heal bruises. A brew can also be used to steam the face to put colour into a pale complexion. Use 250 ml (1 cup) seeds and leaves to a litre (4 cups) boiling water. Boil for 5 minutes. Cool and strain.

CARNATION (*Dianthus caryophyllus*)

Carnation petals can be made into an aromatic vinegar for the bath to ease muscle tension.

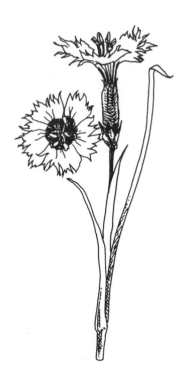

CARROT (*Daucus carota*)

A natural and excellent antiseptic, grated carrot can be applied to skin blemishes and abrasions. Mashed cooked carrots make an amazing drawing poultice and freshly grated carrots added to homemade soaps tone and cleanse the skin. Include fresh carrots frequently in the diet.

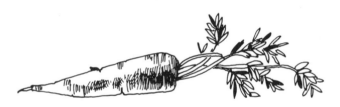

CASTOR OIL PLANT (*Ricinus communis*)

Castor oil can be used externally as a lotion for skin blemishes and itches, or rubbed into eyebrows to make them shine and onto eyelashes to make them grow. As a bath oil, steeped with herbs, it is one of the few oils that disperses and it leaves the skin beautifully soft. As it is a strong purgative, if rubbed into the skin too often it may have a laxative effect, so take care when using it as a massage oil.

CATNIP (*Nepeta cataria*)

Catnip made into a tea – 60 ml (¼ cup) herb to 125–250 ml (½–1 cup) boiling water – is useful for treating bags under the eyes. Apply on wads of cotton-wool. It soothes and reduces swelling, and is also useful rubbed into the scalp to treat dandruff.

CELERY (*Apium graveolens*)

Celery leaves made into a tea and used as a steam or wash have a beautifully toning effect on the skin. I use fresh celery as a bath bag, rubbing well into the skin.

CHAMOMILE (*Anthemis nobilis*)

Make a strong tea (250 ml (1 cup) leaves and flowers to 500 ml–1 litre (2–4 cups) boiling water) and use as a wash to reduce puffiness around the eyes. Dab on frequently with cotton-wool and use as a compress over the eyes. It also relieves general weariness – drink 60 ml (¼ cup) herb to 250 ml (1 cup) boiling water. Use any leftover tea in the bath.

CINNAMON (*Cinnamomum zeylanicum*)

This spice has astringent properties and makes a fragrant addition to hair rinses, softening and giving a rich tone to the hair.

CLOVE (*Caryophyllus aromaticus*)

Chew one or two cloves to sweeten the breath. Make a strong tea (60 ml (¼ cup) cloves to 1 litre (4 cups) boiling water) and use in the bath as an antiseptic wash. Make a weak tea (4 cloves to 125 ml (½ cup) boiling water) and use as an eyewash for tired, sore, red eyes.

COMFREY (*Symphytum officinale*)

Comfrey is a most precious plant in medicine and in cosmetics. It is a cell regenerator and helps to revitalise ageing skins and tissue. It can be used in lotions, creams, salves or ointments and it is always healing and astringent, soothing and antiseptic.

CUCUMBER (*Cucumis sativus*)

Cucumber is extremely useful as a cosmetic as it tightens and tones the skin. It soothes, cools and heals sunburn, windburn and sore eyes (a slice placed on the lids of the eyes for 10 minutes will do wonders to bring back the sparkle). Useful to fade freckles, smooth wrinkles, bleach skin and soften hard skin, cucumber can be made into creams, ointments, soaps, masks and packs. As a bonus, it is also soothing as an after-shave – merely rub a slice or two over the shaved area.

DANDELION (*Taraxacum officinale*)

Dandelions are filled with nourishment, good for skin, liver and urinary systems, and therefore excellent for keeping the skin clear. Make a tea of leaves and flowers – 125 ml (½ cup) herb to 750 ml (3 cups) boiling water – and use as a wash for skin itch, eczema and red skin. Use as a wash for the face as well to invigorate the skin. Steep leaves and flowers in oil and use as a bath or body oil.

ELDER (*Sambucus nigra*)

Flowers, leaves, stems and roots of the elder can all be used medicinally. For cosmetics, though, the flowers are usually used. They are gently astringent and they soothe and soften the skin. Make a tea or wash by pouring 1 litre (4 cups) boiling water over 500 ml (2 cups) flowers. Stand, steep, cool and strain. Keep what you don't use at once in the refrigerator. The leaves make an excellent tea – take equal quantities of water and leaves and boil them up together for 5 minutes, then cool and strain – which can be used to soothe sunburned skin, or give relief from mosquito bites. Diluted, it can be used in the bath and to bleach freckles. Add flowers to night creams and steep in sweet oil for massage.

EUCALYPTUS (*Eucalyptus globulus*)

The leaves of the gum tree make a good bath additive and, if you can find it, the leaves of the lemon scented gum tree are especially beautiful. Add it to creams, oils and vinegars for a wonderful lemon fragrance. An oil made by steeping the leaves in either maize or almond oil makes a soothing rub for aching muscles. A steam for opening and cleansing pores can also be made by pouring a litre (4 cups) boiling water over a bowl packed with leaves. Use a towel tent and inhale – it clears the nose and sinuses too.

FENNEL (*Foeniculum vulgare*)

An infusion of fennel leaves (125 ml (½ cup) herb to 500 ml (2 cups) boiling water) makes an excellent eye bath and is said to have a strengthening effect on the eyes. Fennel tea is a deep cleanser, externally and internally (60 ml (¼ cup) herb to 250 ml (1 cup) boiling water), and is also a diuretic, excellent for those who wish to lose weight.

71

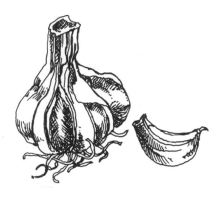

GARLIC (*Allium sativum*)

Garlic is one of nature's wonder herbs. A natural antibiotic, it is a cure for many ailments. For stimulating hair growth infuse 4–6 cloves of garlic, lightly crushed, in 1 litre (4 cups) vinegar and rub into the scalp daily. Use the freshly squeezed juice to dab onto acne or pimples. The only problem is its smell – chew a sprig or two of parsley to get rid of garlic breath.

GERANIUM (*Pelargonium graveolens*)

Scented geraniums (*not the common red geranium*) are soothing and useful in cosmetics, particularly where an astringent is needed. They make wonderful facial steams, and in the bath I find scented geraniums pure pleasure. Use geranium tea – 250 ml (1 cup) herb to 1 litre (4 cups) boiling water – as a face wash, for rinsing the hair or to soothe sunburn. Put a bunch of the leaves next to your bed and bruise them with your fingers from time to time – they'll help you unwind!

GINGER (*Zingiber officinale*)

The fresh rhizome or root of ginger, available at most supermarkets, is a wonderful mouthwash. Take a few thinly shaved pieces, 1–3 teaspoons, and pour over them a cup of boiling water; stand, steep and use as a cleansing and freshening mouthwash.

GRAPES (*Vitis vinifera*)

Grapes are cooling, demulcent and cleansing. Mashed grapes (pips removed) can be applied directly to the skin for a nourishing, skin tightening mask. Leaves added to the bath are restorative and help combat fatigue. Include grapes frequently in your diet as they are cleansing, nourishing and revitalising.

HELIOTROPE (*Heliotropium peruvianum*)

Heliotrope is a favourite fragrant flower in the garden. Its flowers made into a brew – 500 ml (2 cups) flowers to 1 litre (4 cups) boiling water – are a wonderfully invigorating wash and can be added to the bathwater too. Steep the flowers in sunflower oil and use their oil as a bath or massage oil to soothe aching muscles.

HOLLYHOCK (*Althaea rosea*)

Use hollyhock flowers as a rinse for white hair to remove the yellowish tinge. Warm flowers in hot water and apply to the face as a soothing emollient compress for dry flaky skin. Fill a bath bag or add flowers to the bath to treat dry skin.

HONEYSUCKLE (*Lonicera* species)

Gloriously fragrant honeysuckle flowers added to an oil, eg sweet oil or almond oil, make a beautiful massage or body oil. A tea made from flowers and leaves – 500 ml (2 cups) herb to 1 litre (4 cups) boiling water – makes an excellent hair rinse and a wash for delicate skin. If used frequently it helps to smoothe out wrinkles.

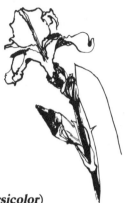

IRIS (*Iris versicolor*)

The exquisite flowers of the iris can be made into a tea – 4 flowers to 500 ml (2 cups) boiling water – which can be used as a cleansing wash for acne and pimples. It cleans and tones the skin and, if used daily, will keep the skin oil and spot free. Use this same brew as a rinse for oily hair. Infuse iris flowers in sweet oil and use as a massage oil for aching legs and cramps.

IVY (*Hedera helix*)

A leaf soaked overnight in salt and vinegar and applied to a corn (a fresh leaf bound in place each night) will soften and remove the corn. Use an ivy and geranium leaf mixture in the bath. Boil up 500 ml (2 cups) ivy leaves in 1 litre (4 cups) water for 5 minutes and apply as a sunburn soother.

JASMINE (*Jasminum officinale*)

The beautiful highly fragrant jasmine, infused in white vinegar, makes a glorious bath vinegar, which, dabbed onto aching feet, will also soothe and smooth. Made into an oil (use almond or sweet oil), jasmine makes a perfect massage oil and soothing body oil. I make a huge quantity in spring and use it as a bath oil all through winter. Flowers made into a tea are said to be aphrodisiac!

LAVENDER (*Lavandula officinalis, L. spica*)

A beloved herb, lavender is one of the most well-used herbs in cosmetics. Make a strong lavender oil by infusing flowers and leaves in a good oil, eg sweet oil, and use as a rub for aching muscles, or in the bath for softening the skin. Lavender vinegar can be brushed and rubbed into the hair to stimulate hair growth and, rubbed onto the temples, will soothe fatigue and headaches. Have a bunch of lavender leaves and flowers at the bedside and touch and bruise them from time to time – the fragrance will help you sleep. Lavender tea – 60 ml (¼ cup) herb to 250 ml (1 cup) boiling water – relieves exhaustion and will help you unwind. This same brew is an excellent face wash and a stronger brew can be rubbed into the hair – 250 ml (1 cup) herb to 250 ml (1 cup) boiling water – to stimulate hair growth. Dab it onto pimples and acne, or use as a gargle to freshen the mouth. You can splash it on as an aftershave lotion or use it in bath oils, vinegars, soaps and perfumes.

LEMON (*Citrus limon*)

Lemon is an aromatic astringent and is used in many ways. Add the fresh peel to your bath to soften the skin, and the juice to the rinsing water after you have shampooed your hair. Use diluted juice as a rinse for oily skin, as a face wash and as a freshener. Dig your nails into a squeezed lemon to strengthen and cleanse them. Rub a halved, squeezed lemon over rough heels and elbows. Drink lemon juice in hot water or herb teas daily to keep the skin clear. Dab the juice onto spots and blemishes.

LEMON BALM (*Melissa officinalis*)

This lemony mint is best used fresh, made into a tea – 250 ml (1 cup) lemon balm leaves to 750 ml (3 cups) boiling water – for an excellent face or hair wash. It can also be used in the bath or drunk as a reviving tea. It heals and cleanses blemished skin, and, drunk as a tea, also helps lift depression.

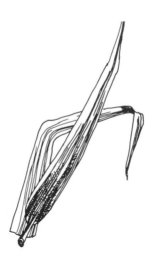

LEMON GRASS (*Cymbopogon citratus*)

This is a most delicious and fragrant grass. It is the fastest selling herb in my herb nursery and the favourite tea of all the students who attend my classes at the Herb Centre. A tea made of the leaves not only makes an excellent cleansing, astringent wash (250 ml (1 cup) leaves to 1 litre (4 cups) boiling water), but added to bathwater, it revives and refreshes. It cleanses oily skin, combats dandruff, spots and blackheads and makes a nice aftershave lotion. It is also soothing to tired feet if splashed on after a bath, and makes a beautiful hair rinse after shampooing.

LEMON VERBENA (*Lippia citriodora*)

This is another beautiful bath herb, richly fragrant, and one of the few herbs that never loses its fragrance when it is dried. It is a pore stimulant and a strong tea, made of 500 ml (2 cups) lemon verbena leaves to 1 litre (4 cups) boiling water, can be used as a steam or as a wash. Dab onto oily skin as a freshener, particularly to patches of acne on the neck and back. Use fresh leaves in a bath glove or bag or make lemon verbena vinegar or oil and use in the bath.

LETTUCE (*Lactuca sativa*)

Ordinary lettuce is an effective wash for pimply skin. Simmer a whole lettuce in enough water to cover it for a few minutes and use the water as a wash. Nursing mothers can dab it onto sore nipples; bathe the breasts in it, too, to give relief. Cooked lettuce, with salt, pepper, a little butter and a squeeze of lemon juice, will increase the milk flow. Lettuce water will soothe sunburn and rough, wind-burned skin.

LUCERNE (*Medicago sativa*)

Lucerne made into a tea is an exfoliant (remember the patch test). The leaves can be made into a tea – 250 ml (1 cup) leaves to 750 ml (3 cups) boiling water – and used as a wash or as a steam. Dabbed frequently onto greasy, pimply areas, it will cleanse and heal. Mix chopped or minced lucerne leaves with pawpaw and apply as a mask – it will gently peel off dry, rough areas. Use lucerne, fresh young and green, in the diet to keep the skin clear, the muscles toned and energy flowing! A great many people in my classes have found it gives them stamina, and are always on the lookout for a patch of lucerne on their travels. Lucerne is also known as alfalfa, and is familiar as a sprouting vegetable.

MARJORAM (*Origanum majorana*)

Marjoram, fresh or dried, can be steeped in oil and used as a soothing rub for bruises, sprains or strains. Use it as a bath oil or vinegar as it stimulates the circulation and is good for the skin.

MAIZE/CORN (*Zea mays*)

The silk from the sweet corn can be ground and finely pounded and used in talc and face powder. Cornflour made from this is useful as a homemade talc and is soothing and smoothing.

MELONS (Cucurbitaceae family)

Most members of this family can be used to make face masks because of their tightening, cleansing and toning properties. The mashed pulp can be added to oatmeal or ground corn flour and made into a mask or poultice. *Watermelon* is particularly cleansing and freshening for oily skin. *Honeydew* or *cantaloup* are good for normal to dry skins. Use melon slices as a compress for tired eyes.

MINTS (*Mentha* species)

Mints are stimulants and there is such a wide variety to choose from that you should easily find one that will please you. From spearmint to orange mint, chocolate mint to eau-de-Cologne mint, apple mint to ginger mint, there is a delicious fragrance for every taste. Combine mint with rosemary vinegar for a good dandruff treatment. Rub a strong mint tea – 250 ml (1 cup) herb to 500 ml (2 cups) boiling water – into the scalp daily to stimulate hair growth. Use this same tea in the bath to stimulate the circulation – you will find it reviving when you are over-tired. Pour boiling water over a bowl of mint leaves and use as a facial steam; it will cleanse and tone the skin and combat oiliness and open pores. Use the tea as a mouth wash, too, or dab onto tired, aching feet. Dip a compress into it and use it to treat a headache.

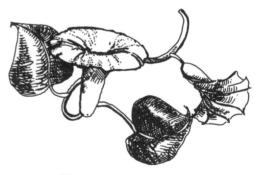

MORNING GLORY (*Ipomoea purpurea*)

The beautiful blue flowers of the morning glory can be used as a compress over tired, sore eyes. Dip 4–6 flowers in hot water, place a couple over the eyes and relax for a few minutes. Then replace those flowers with two more, and so on. Make a strong tea – 250 ml (1 cup) herb to 750 ml (3 cups) boiling water – stand, strain and use as a hair rinse for lustreless hair, rubbing in well.

MYRTLE (*Myrtus communis*)

Myrtle leaves are antiseptic and can be used in a douche – 125 ml (½ cup) leaves boiled up in 750 ml (3 cups) boiling water. Stand, steep, then strain. Use leaves in bath vinegars, gloves, and wash bags. Myrtle is wonderfully refreshing and invigorating.

NASTURTIUM (*Tropaeolum majus*)

Bright nasturtium flowers are excellent used in the bath as an astringent. Use a tea – 250 ml (1 cup) flowers to 500 ml (2 cups) boiling water – as a rinse for golden blonde and red hair. Use leaves and flowers in salads, as they are full of vitamin C. One of nature's antibiotics, nasturtium will also assist in keeping the skin clear.

NETTLE (*Urtica ureus, U. dioica*)

Nettles are wonderful in the bath (pick them with gloves on!) tied into an old stocking. Hot water renders harmless the acid which causes the sting. Use with a good soap to rub all over the skin. Arthritis sufferers find it especially soothing. Made into a tea – 250 ml (1 cup) herb to 750 ml (3 cups) boiling water – nettles can be used as a scalp massage to stimulate hair growth. They can also be infused into vinegar for rubbing into the scalp. Nettles have a centuries-old reputation as a blood purifier. Made into a spinach, they make a delicious meal and help to clear skins as well.

NUTMEG (*Myristica fragrans*)

Stand several nutmegs that have been roughly cracked in sweet oil for 3 weeks. Strain and use this oil as a rub for aching legs and heels, and over aching joints. Nutmeg stimulates the circulation and soothes aches and pains, particularly those resulting from physical exercise.

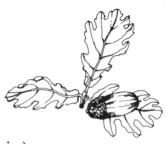

OAK (*Quercus* species)

Oak leaves and bark are mildly antiseptic and, mixed with mint or comfrey, make a good antiseptic wash for grazes and skin eruptions, and can be used as a mouthwash too.

OATS (*Avena sativa*)

Oats are a useful ingredient in cosmetics as they are deep cleansing, softening and soothing. Make a thin oats porridge to rub onto insect bites and scratches after a day in the veld. Allow to dry, then rinse off in a bath. Rub more oats into the skin while bathing. Oats are also good for nappy rash, and raw oats, mixed with honey or yoghurt, make an excellent facial, chest and back scrub. Add oats to soaps and bath bags, or rub into hands to soften and cleanse. Use oats frequently – they are a natural cosmetic. (I find the large-flake, non-instant kind the best.)

OLIVE (*Olea europaea*)

A rich and heavy oil, medicinal olive oil can be added to bathwater, soap and, combined with other oils, for massage. Steep chamomile flowers, rosemary and lemon peel in olive oil for a deep soothing and softening effect. Use as a cuticle oil and to rub into cracks in the heels and around the toes. Combined with vitamin E and a little coconut oil, it can be used to fade stretch-marks; massage in each evening.

ORANGES (*Citrus* species)

The familiar orange has many uses. Orange blossom is invigorating in vinegar used in bath bags, and the peel can be dried and added to bath vinegar and hair rinses. The leaves can be used in bath gloves and wash bags and have a stimulating effect. Add fresh flowers to creams and lotions as an enriching agent – especially good for ageing, dry skins. Try making your own orange flower water by filling a jar with orange blossom, one or two leaves and a twist of peel. Fill with vodka and leave for 3 weeks, shaking the jar every now and then. Pour off a little and dilute with water in a 1:10 ratio and use as an astringent or freshener.

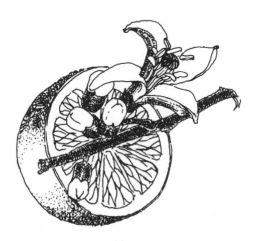

ORIGANUM (*Origanum vulgare*)

This is a soothing herb to use in the bath to ease aching muscles. Make origanum oil by steeping sprigs of origanum in sweet oil or sunflower oil, and add it to the bathwater. This same oil can be rubbed into an itchy scalp for quick relief.

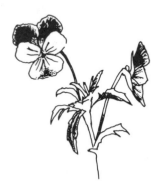 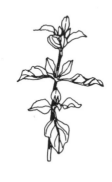

PANSY (*Viola tricolor*)

The beautiful little pansy or heart's ease, which brightens up winter gardens, is a very useful herb for skin and hair. It contains salicylic acid, which makes it a soothing, astringent herb. Use it in baths, lotions, vinegars, creams and ointments. It is an excellent wash for eczema and for cradle cap in babies – 250 ml (1 cup) flowers and leaves to 500 ml–1 litre (2–4 cups) boiling water. Fresh leaves can be rubbed onto pimples and they will soothe and cool the inflammation.

PARSLEY (*Petroselinum crispum*)

Eat parsley daily for fresh breath. Parsley cleanses the kidneys, thus keeping the skin clear and the eyes sparkling. Parsley tea is medicinal and cleansing – 250 ml (1 cup) herb to 750 ml (3 cups) boiling water. Dab this tea onto eczema, psoriasis and skin irritations and you will find it wonderfully helpful.

PAWPAW (*Carica papaya*)

This is another of nature's wonder plants. Mash the flesh and apply it as a mask to cleanse greasy skin. The seeds can be mashed and mixed with oatmeal to make a deep cleansing treatment for blemished and oily complexions. The milk from the stems is an exfoliant but dilute and test it very well before using. The leaves, too, can be chopped and applied as an exfoliant. Mix them with borage or comfrey leaves and include them in the diet. Pawpaw keeps the bowels regular and the skin clear and bright.

PEA (*Pisum sativum*)

Fresh garden peas contain vitamin E. Cooked and mashed, they can be applied to varicose veins and haemorrhoids. They are soothing and contracting, and the water in which they are cooked makes an excellent wash for all skin types.

PEACH (*Prunus persica*)

Use peach leaves in the bath as an emollient. They can also be added to facial masks for normal or dry skins. A fresh, skinned peach makes an excellent mask for sunburned skins, and the peach kernels, boiled up in apple cider vinegar for 5 minutes and then left to cool, will stimulate hair growth if rubbed daily onto the scalp.

PEAR (*Pyrus communis*)

Ripe mashed pear is a cooling, soothing application for sunburn. A slice of pear laid over tired eyes is very relaxing and soothing, and mashed, ripe pear flesh makes an excellent face mask for normal skin. Smooth on and allow to dry slightly for 15-20 minutes. Wash off with tepid water.

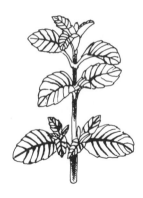

PENNYROYAL (*Mentha pulegium*)

This is a wonderful bath herb as it is stimulating and invigorating and soothes dry, itchy skin. Make a strong tea – 250 ml (1 cup) herb to 250–500 ml (1–2 cups) boiling water – and rub onto the skin as a deodorant.

PERIWINKLE (*Vinca major, V. minor*)

Periwinkle is excellent when made into an astringent wash (250 ml (1 cup) herb to 750 ml (3 cups) boiling water) for skin irritations and blemishes. It is an old-fashioned beauty aid, well known for many years. I use the leaves in bath bags to soothe scratches and abrasions after a day in the outdoors. Fresh, boiled leaves make an excellent wash for cradle cap.

PINE (*Pinus* species)

Pine-needles make a wonderfully stimulating addition to the bath as they are deodorising, freshening and soothe aches and pains. Best of all, as a 'wake-up' bath in the morning, put pine-needles in the water (I use them in gloves and in bath bags) to invigorate and cleanse. A strong pine-needle tea can also be made as an after-shower splash-on – 6 cups pine-needles boiled up in 3 litres (12 cups) boiling water. Use this brew, too, as an aftershave and as an under-arm deodorant.

PINEAPPLE (*Ananas sativus*)

The juice and flesh of the common pineapple make an excellent astringent wash for oily and blemished skin. It also acts as an exfoliant and the juice makes a good gargle for sore throats.

POMEGRANATE (*Punica granatum*)

The juice of the pomegranate is a very good astringent for oily skin. It deep cleanses and closes the pores. It is a slight skin dye, too, and gives a warm glow to the skin. It also acts as an internal cleanser, so include it in your diet to keep your skin looking good.

POTATO (*Solanum tuberosum*)

Raw sliced potato placed on bruises will soon soothe them and remove discoloration. Raw potato is also excellent for stopping itchiness and dryness as it contains potassium which works quickly. It will even relieve nettle stings, scratches and insect bites.

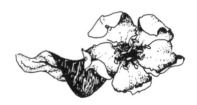

QUINCE (*Cydonia oblongata*)

One of my favourite herbs, the quince is excellent for encouraging luxurious, shiny hair growth. Make a strong brew from peels, cores and skins, boiled up, then cooled and strained. Comb into the hair daily. Grated quince flesh, with oats, is an excellent scrub to cleanse grey, dirty skin. Quince tea, made from flesh, peel and leaves and added to the bathwater, will tone and revive aching muscles.

ROSE (*Rosa* species)

Perhaps the most loved of all flowers, rose petals, boiled up in water (enough to cover the petals) make a beautiful rosewater. Add equal quantities vodka or cane spirit if you want it to keep. Make rose-petal vinegar to use as a deodorant and use rose petals in sweet oil for baths, massages and rubs.

ROSEMARY (*Rosmarinus officinalis*)

Rosemary is a herb with so many uses, you should always have a bush in your garden. It is a healing, astringent herb, very good for skin and hair. It can be made into a tea – 250 ml (1 cup) herb to 250–500 ml (1–2 cups) boiling water – and used as a hair rinse, facial wash, a gargle, scalp treatment or, adding a spoon of honey, to revive one after a hard day! Make rosemary oil, rosemary vinegar, or rosemary soap.

SAGE (*Salvia officinalis*)

Make sage tea – 250 ml (1 cup) herb to 500 ml (2 cups) boiling water – to massage into the hair to cleanse and tone the scalp and darken the hair. The same brew will heal spots and blemishes if used as a wash, and in the bath it will stimulate blood circulation to the skin. Used as an under-arm wash, it is a refreshing deodorant.

ST JOHN'S WORT (*Hypericum perforatum*)

Infuse the bright yellow flowers of hypericum in sweet oil, or sunflower or maize oil. Use as a rub for tired and aching muscles. Make a tea, using 750 ml (3 cups) flowers to 500 ml (2 cups) boiling water, and add it to shampoo. It will give lustre to lifeless hair, particularly after a long illness.

SNAPDRAGON (*Antirrhinum majus*)

Steep snapdragon flowers in castor oil or almond oil, and use as a salve for bruises or haemorrhoids and as a rub for irritated skin. Use fresh flowers in bath bags to soothe chafed skin. Snapdragon tea, 60 ml (¼ cup) flowers to 250 ml (1 cup) boiling water, is said to improve the sense of taste!

SOAPWORT (*Saponaria officinalis*)

Boil up a big pot of soapwort leaves, stems, roots and flowers, in just enough water to cover. Stand and steep for half an hour, then strain. Use this soapy brew to wash freshly shampooed hair; it will revitalise heat-damaged, permed, dyed or bleached hair. Use also as a wash or to dab onto eczema, skin rashes and heat rash. It is also good for nappy rash. Use as a weekly hair conditioner to restore lustre to the hair.

SOUTHERNWOOD (*Artemisia abrotanum*)

Boil up 500 ml (2 cups) southernwood leaves with 125 ml (½ cup) barley in 1 litre (4 cups) water for half an hour (simmer with the lid on). Strain and use as a wash for pimples and acne. Make a strong tea – 250 ml (1 cup) herb to 250 ml (1 cup) boiling water – and rub into the scalp (or beard) to stimulate growth.

SOW'S THISTLE (*Sonchus oleraceus*)

This common weed contains a milky juice that can be effectively applied to pimples. It dries them up and heals, removing the redness. A tea made of leaves, flowers and stems (250 ml (1 cup) herb to 250 ml (1 cup) boiling water) is an excellent wash for spotty skins. Eat some young leaves in salads, too, to keep the skin clear.

STRAWBERRY (*Fragaria vesca*)

Strawberry leaves make an excellent astringent wash and, used in the bath, are particularly good for oily skins. Brew up 250 ml (1 cup) leaves to 750 ml (3 cups) boiling water, stand, steep and cool. Use ripe, mashed fruit as a face pack – it is astringent and tightening. Combine with oats or ground corn flour as a cleansing and invigorating face pack for oily skin and coarse pores.

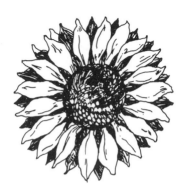

SUNFLOWER (*Helianthus annuus*)

Ground sunflower seeds make an excellent nutritious face pack. Grind 500 ml (2 cups) seeds and mix with milk for dry skins and yoghurt for oily skins, to form a paste. Apply to a clean, damp face and allow it to dry (I find 20 minutes is about the time needed – relax and read a book). Wash off with warm water. Use sunflower petals in hair rinses for blonde hair.

TANSY (*Tanacetum vulgare*)

Tansy is a cleanser – make a tea of 250 ml (1 cup) leaves to 750 ml (3 cups) boiling water, stand, steep for 20 minutes and strain. Dab onto pimples and use as a wash. Combine this herb with comfrey or chamomile flowers.

TEA (*Thea sinensis*)

A cooled, used teabag makes an effective poultice for soothing sunburn. Place a wet bag over the eyes to reduce puffiness or to use as a compress for headaches or over-tired eyes.

THYME (*Thymus vulgaris*)

Thyme is antiseptic and stimulant. A thyme tea – 250 ml (1 cup) herb to 750 ml (3 cups) boiling water – is an effective under-arm deodorant, aftershave lotion, mouth and face wash for problem skins, or a deep cleanser. Use it in the bath, in vinegar as a hair rinse and as a face steam. Apply the tea to eczema, psoriasis and rashes.

TUBEROSE (*Polianthes tuberosa*)

The gloriously fragrant flowers of the tuberose can be steeped in oil (preferably sweet oil or almond oil) and used as a massage oil or in the bath. Vinegar made with tuberoses (see section on vinegars) has a beautiful, lingering fragrance.

VANILLA (*Vanilla planifolia*)

The beans of the vanilla vine should be treasured, as, infused in oil, they can be used over and over again. Vanilla is soothing and smoothing to the skin, and in bath oil (I like almond oil best) vanilla is a treat.

VERBASCUM (Mullein) (*Verbascum thapsus*)

The leaves and flowers of verbascum are used wherever astringent or emollient properties are needed. It is excellent for hair rinses, especially for oily hair: 500 ml (2 cups) leaves and flowers to 750 ml (3 cups) boiling water. Stand for 20 minutes, strain and use. A thick decoction of flowers, boiled up, makes a yellow hair dye. Steep the flowers in oil and use as a massage oil for aching muscles.

VETIVER (Khus-khus grass) (*Vetiveria zizanioides*)

The highly fragrant root of the mature vetiver grass can be used in oil or in vinegar. It makes a beautiful addition to bath-water and is soothing and softening. The oil is also an enriching, soothing massage oil.

VIOLET (*Viola odorata*)

The leaves and flowers of the common garden violet are emollient and soothing. They can be made into a tea: use 250 ml (1 cup) flowers and leaves to 500 ml (2 cups) boiling water, stand for half an hour, then strain. Use this tea for skin irritations, spotty skin, rash, sunburn or wind-burn. Violet water is a soothing aftershave lotion and as a dab onto a baby's chafed skin, or for nappy rash. In a double boiler simmer the leaves and flowers in almond oil, add lanolin and use as a soothing lotion for dry skin.

WALNUT (*Juglans nigra*)

Walnut hulls, boiled up in water, make a dark brown hair or skin dye. A decoction of leaves (500 ml (2 cups) leaves to 750 ml–1,5 litres (3–6 cups) boiling water) can be added to shampoos and hair rinses or used in the bath as an invigorating astringent. A stronger brew is said to be soothing and healing when dabbed onto skin eruptions such as herpes; used as a mouthwash, it clears up minor mouth infections. Steep leaves and hulls in oil and use as a scalp massage to clear dandruff.

WATERCRESS (*Nasturtium officinale*)

Watercress is astringent and cleansing. Use fresh in a bath bag for blemishes and freckles. Make a strong tea – 250 ml (1 cup) watercress to 250 ml (1 cup) boiling water, and dab onto freckles and spots, or use as a wash.